CHEF ANDREA DRUMMER

T0098759

CANNABIS CUISINE

Bud Pairings of A Born Again Chef

Cover + Layout Design : Elina Diaz
Author Photo: Jack Sheldon

For permission requests, please contact the publisher at:

Mango Publishing Group
2850 Douglas Road, 3rd Floor
Coral Gables, FL 33134 USA
info@mango.bz

For special orders, quantity sales, course adoptions and corporate sales, please email the publisher at sales@mango.bz. For trade and wholesale sales, please contact Ingram Publisher Services at customer.service@ingramcontent.com or +1.800.509.4887.

Cannabis Cuisine: Bud Pairings of A Born Again Chef

Library of Congress Cataloging
ISBN: 978-1-63353-667-8, (ebook) 978-1-63353-668-5
Library of Congress Control Number: 2017913089
BISAC category code: CKB040000 COOKING / Specific Ingredients / Herbs, Spices, Condiments
CKB059000 COOKING / Specific Ingredients / Natural Foods

Printed in the United States of America

My father said that he took risks because he had children to care for.
I always thought that he took risks because he was superman.
Whatever the matter, from him I learned to be fearless.

From my mother, I learned other lessons: to cook, to love, to pray,
to forgive, to laugh out loud and often at one's self.

From them both, I've learned to relish balance.

CONTENTS

PREFACE

I tried cannabis for the first time in junior high school. I remember the "friend" who offered it to me. I remember the feather-ended roach clip that held the joint, which was certainly long enough to smoke without. I recall the acrid smell of the smoke I released from the one long pull, the dizzying sensation, and the feeling of being out of sync with my own thoughts. I was high and I didn't like it.

My frustration made me rash. I demanded to be returned to the school that I had ditched for the day. "Maybe you should just sleep it off, and I'll take you home later," the friend suggested. By now, though, I no longer trusted him or myself. I was having trouble harnessing my thoughts and hoped being in a familiar and safe environment would reverse the effects. How wrong I was.

Against his better judgment, he returned me to Parkway Middle School just in time for my last class of the day. Within five minutes of being on campus, my discomfort and paranoia got the better of me. I incited a fight with a friend and ally. Not just a verbal assault but a physical altercation that sent her to the hospital and me to court. Suffice to say, it was a sobering experience.

I was sentenced to 200 hours of community service in exchange for an expunged record, which is why I spent that summer at a consignment shop whose proceeds benefitted a shelter for victims of domestic violence. My sympathetic female supervisors initially stuck me in the clothes section, thinking I might like getting first pick of the offerings. But when they realized I liked to read, they assigned me to the book section in the back. Consequently, I literally read my way through those 200 hours, and it was there that I came upon one book that really resonated with me. It was "Go Ask Alice," the diary of a teenage drug-addicted girl. I was convinced that if I ever tried marijuana again, her horrific life would be mine.

I reference this incident because it was an integral part of my journey from cannabis paranoia to writing about cannabis pairings. I believed then that all cannabis had the same effect and would result in death or prison. This idea was reinforced by the church and by the Reagan administration's anti-drug campaign. It gave me permission to judge others and declare myself a martyr. I preached the gospel for many years, counseling young and old about the perilous road of cannabis use. Without much knowledge of the marijuana plant, I, like many Americans, demonized it and anyone subscribed to it.

I was wrong.

What I didn't know was that the strain of cannabis that I smoked that first day was likely grown under duress and in ill circumstances. I didn't know then that cannabis not only has different strains, but also differs depending on how it was produced and who is using it. That particular strain just may not have suited me. I knew nothing of the flavor profiles, indicas versus sativas, hybrids, the varied effects, or of CBD or its many medicinal properties.

Perhaps you, like me, judged. Perhaps you do still. But maybe, just maybe...you too can be born again.

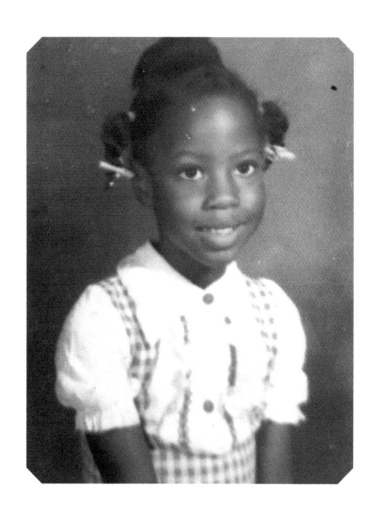

INTRODUCTION

Every chef gets the question at least once...a month: What's your favorite dish to cook?

To this day, I'm at a loss for words. I rally my most diplomatic face and launch into a pseudo – intellectual rant about not being pigeonholed, the value of exploration, and blah, blah, blah, but in fact, I feel like indignantly asking a few questions in return: Would you ask a painter which painting he likes most to paint? Or an architect which building he most likes to design? You see, while the technique is generally applicable, the art and joy is in rediscovering; it's in challenging one's ability to the beyond. The true answer to the ubiquitous question is my favorite thing to cook is food.

The seeds of becoming a chef were sown long before I could understand what was happening. They were planted at my inception and cultivated through family and life experiences. Sometimes just a small thing can enter your life and change you profoundly and forever: a great bottle of wine, a child, an idea—for me, it was the moment that I realized the endless possibilities of food and its preparation. I am not speaking only of the skilled choreography that it takes to bring a culinary idea to life, or the intricate melding of spices, products, and protein. I'm speaking also of the universal role that food has in bringing people together to love, share ideas, laugh and...well, just be. To prepare food is to introduce an idea—it is the taste of sun in a peach or the saline flavor of an oyster that dances on the back of your palette. The possibilities of food forced my hand in every regard and shaped a career that was predestined.

I remember the day I discovered a tomato for the first time. It wasn't the first time I had eaten a tomato, but this time I discovered it; it was unveiled to me in all of its authenticity. My cousin and I (at six and seven years old) snuck into our grandmother's garden and pillaged a few vine-ripened tomatoes. We scurried into the bathroom having quickly swiped the saltshaker. There, for the first time I came to understand the nuances of a tomato. I inwardly marveled at the texture of the flesh as it differed from the skin. I lapped up the seeds and pulp, feeling the texture and bite with my teeth. I noticed the taste changed depending on how much salt I used.

These overt and subtle differences in flavor and texture piqued my interest. I was learning not only to explore food but also to dissect it. I was learning the difference between simply eating a carrot and unearthing the change in flavor between the core and root of the vegetable. I studied the taste, texture, and density of peanuts, almonds, or pecans, as I ate them one by one, in four to six bites per single nut.

This concept alone led me through masses of people on a Sunday afternoon, in search of the best sea bass or scallops or salmon or duck in Philadelphia's 9th Street Italian Market. Years later, it engrossed me in the food markets of New York's Chinatown—fish flying in midair, buyers prying, barterers shouting, and early morning onlookers gaping. And now, the same concept, with an even greater pull as of music wafting from a magic pipe, beckons me again, leading me through rows of the freshest produce at Los Angeles's farmers markets.

As I look beyond the crowd, in search of the best locally grown mushrooms and pea tendrils, I always keep my eye out for something else: inspiration! I pick up a piece of fruit and ask what it would like to become. I eat the flesh of blood orange samples, nibble the rind, and breathe in the scent of its zest. While bagging the best quality of chanterelles, I consider them at their finest hour, tasting the stems, the caps, and the gills. I consider a particular impending dining experience. I'm careful to honor the integrity of the product.

Finally we arrive to the present, where I've gleefully brought in an exciting new concept and ingredient to the repertoire—cannabis. But wait, it is actually no different from the fresh corn that my father used to bestow upon us as kids, or the ripened berries, peaches, and crab apples that we'd pick along the roadside. I dissect cannabis as I do everything else: carefully and consideringly. I smell and taste its potential as a full-bodied ingredient, honoring the integrity of the various strains and perfectly pairing them with other ingredients, flavors, textures, and tastes.

Obviously one of my favorite things about cooking is the creativity which goes into it: the inspiration behind it, the thoughtfulness of its design, the equilibrium of the served dishes, the careful balance within the ingredients, and the smell of the menu coming together. But one aspect of this process that moves me beyond creativity is the discovery, the exploration, and the infinite possibilities of the process.

Long before this process became my calling, I held the belief that the presentation should be the voice where there are no words. There is magnificence to a project when it takes effort and care to pull together. (Like the extra arch of a brow, or the matching lingerie of lovers; the perfect shade of red lipstick or a heel just high enough that he notices it but still feels empowered.) Every detail of flavor and presentation joins in a grand symphony of piquancy, placed with the deft hand of an artist. This is what I bring to every person who encounters my food or dines with me at a dinner party—the undeniable sense that I care deeply not only about my ingredients, but also about you, the diner.

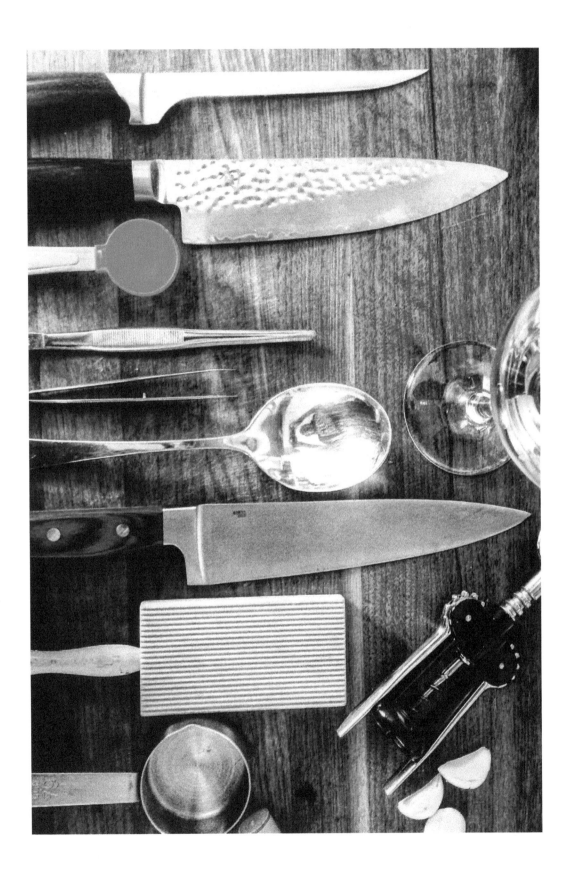

FUNDAMENTALS

The Food

To cultivate a great bud strain, one must first identify and then procure a seed of choice. The seed must be sown with great consideration to the climate and the soil. And finally, careful attention must be given to the growing process. Partner that with produce, meats, and cheeses that have been given the same consideration and you have the beginnings of a masterful culinary experience one can be proud of.

The Event

To orchestrate a great dining experience, one must first identify the participants of choice. The menu items must be chosen with great consideration to time and place. And finally, careful attention must be given to the orchestration of the whole.

These are the fundamentals.

CALCULATING THC

One of the major differences between edible consumption of the past and the present is dosage control. The sophisticated consumer now has the ability to create an elite foundation of oils and butters with specific THC calculations, resulting in a consumable meal without angst.

The scientific determination of THC levels is calculated with basic math and the knowledge of any cannabis product (i.e. Bud, Shake, Trim). Knowing the present levels of THC is what makes the difference between having a great edible experience and shying away in fear, as many first-time consumers do. I was one of those consumers.

I have specific purveyors for my cannabis materials. I get my fish on Fridays and my produce on Wednesdays, because that is when my specialists are selling. These suppliers are well versed in their craft; they know their products—the THC levels of each; the flavor profiles of each. Their interest and acumen reassure me that I will consistently receive the best quality produce from them. We are a team. And we invite you, the consumer, to join us.

This is the first and most important recipe in your arsenal.

HOW TO CALCULATE

*FOR EASE OF DEMONSTRATING HOW TO USE THE FORMULA I WILL USE A THC LEVEL OF 10%

Convert your cannabis from grams to milligrams.

- 28.3 grams is approximately equal to 1 ounce

- 28.3 grams x 1,000 equals 28,300 milligrams of THC.

- 28,300 x 10% (THC level) equals 2,830 mg of THC per batch.

2830 divided by 32 Tbsp. (1 pound of butter) equals 88.4 mg of THC per Tbsp. of butter.

To determine the dosage level per serving, take the total number of THC your dish has and divide by the number of servings it yields.

At the above levels (88.4 mg THC), if your dish calls for 1 Tbsp. of butter and yields 6 servings, then your THC level per serving would be about 14 mg per serving (88.4/6).

There are several apps and websites available that will calculate the THC levels of your material with greater ease: https://www.whaxy.com/calculatorhttps://www.jeffthe420chef.com/calculator

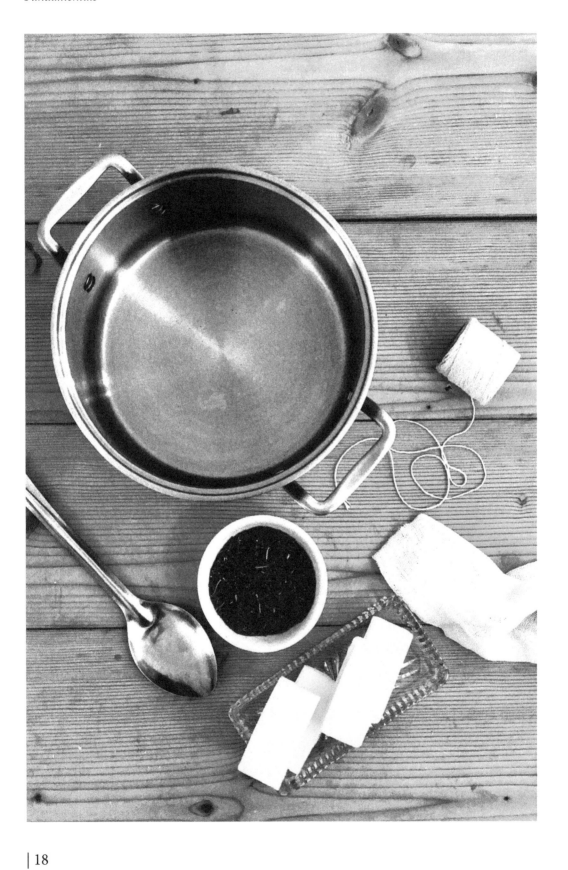

CLARIFIED BUTTER

1 lb. of unsalted butter

INSTRUCTIONS

Place the butter in a 2-quart saucepan and set over medium heat.

Once the butter has melted, lower the heat to lowest setting and then adjust to maintain a low boil.

Cook for approximately 45 minutes, until butter is clear, and foam on top is slightly browned.

Strain the clarified butter using a chinois or layered cheesecloth set into a strainer.

Butter should be clear and devoid of all milk fat.

CLEAN CANNABIS BUTTER

YIELDS 212 MG OF THC PER TBSP.

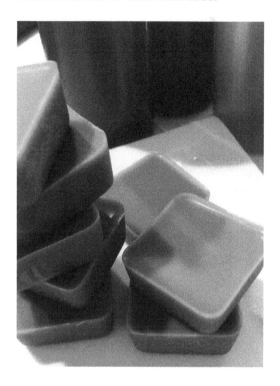

28.3 grams of cannabis product (1 ounce)
1 lb. of unsalted clarified butter (reference recipe)
Cheesecloth
Cooking grade cotton twine

INSTRUCTIONS

Grind cannabis material, using a coffee grinder or blender.

Place material in layered cheesecloth, creating a sachet. Secure tightly with cooking grade cotton twine.

Add the sachet to melted clarified butter

in a 2-quart saucepan.

Place over low heat and cook for 3 hours to extract the THC content from the material, thereby infusing the clarified butter.

Stir occasionally to prevent scorching of the butter.

Do not allow the butter to come to a boil.

Strain the final product using a chinois or layered cheesecloth set into a strainer placed over a heat resistant receptacle. Allow to cool fully before refrigerating.

*Keeps for up to 1 year.

**Recipes based on Clean Cannabis Butter made with product containing between 22 – 24% THC.

ROASTED GARLIC & CHIVE BUTTER

YIELDS 8 MG OF THC PER TBSP.

*8 Tbsp. (1 stick) of unsalted butter
(room temperature)*

*1 tsp. of clean cannabis butter
(room temperature)*

*1 head of roasted garlic
(reference recipe)*

*2 ½ Tbsp. of chives
(blanched and chopped)*

Pinch of salt

Plastic wrap

TO ROAST THE GARLIC:

Slice the top off 1 head of garlic.
Drizzle with olive oil, wrap in foil, and roast at 400 degrees. Cook until tender, cool, and then squeeze out cloves.

INSTRUCTIONS

Smash roasted garlic into a paste along with salt.

Gently fold together butter, Clean Cannabis Butter garlic paste, and chopped chive.

Spoon butter in a cylinder shape into the center of a square of plastic wrap.

Roll into a tight tubular shape, twisting the ends. Refrigerate.

BLACKENED SEASONING BUTTER

YIELDS 8 MG OF THC PER TBSP.

*8 Tbsp. (1 stick) of unsalted butter
(room temperature)*

*1 tsp. of Clean Cannabis Butter
(room temperature)*

1 ½ tsp. dried thyme

1 ½ tsp. dried oregano

½ tsp. cumin

1 tsp. garlic powder

1 tsp. onion powder

¼ tsp. brown sugar

¼ tsp. granulated sugar

¼ tsp. smoked paprika

½ tsp. paprika

¼ tsp. cayenne pepper

¼ tsp. salt

Plastic wrap

INSTRUCTIONS

Mix dry ingredients.

Gently fold together butter, Clean Cannabis Butter, and seasonings.

Spoon butter in a cylinder shape into the center of a square of plastic wrap.

Roll into a tight tubular shape, twisting the ends. Refrigerate.

HONEY ROSE BUTTER

YIELDS 8 MG OF THC PER TBSP.

8 Tbsp. (1 stick) of unsalted butter (room temperature)

1 tsp. of Clean Cannabis Butter (room temperature)

1 tsp. rose water

1 ½ Tbsp. dried edible rose petals

2 ½ Tbsp. honey

Pinch of salt

Plastic wrap

INSTRUCTIONS

Gently mix butter, Clean Cannabis Butter, honey and rose water, and salt until there are no streaks.

Fold in rose petals until evenly distributed.

Spoon butter in a cylinder shape into the center of a square of plastic wrap.

Roll into a tight tubular shape, twisting the ends. Refrigerate.

CANNABIS OIL

YIELDS 141 MG OF THC PER TBSP.

28.3 grams of cannabis product (1 ounce)

32 ounces high temperature canola oil

Cheesecloth

INSTRUCTIONS

Grind cannabis material, using a designated coffee grinder or blender.

Place material in layered cheesecloth, creating a sachet. Secure tightly with cooking grade cotton twine.

Place oil in 4-quart pot over low heat.

Add sachet of cannabis and cook on low heat for up to 1 ½–2 hours.

Stir occasionally. Do not allow oil to arrive at a boiling state.

Allow oil to cool and then strain using a chinois or layered cheesecloth set into a strainer.

For extended shelf life, store in a dark bottle and keep in cool dry place or refrigerator

Note: THC degrades at temperatures exceeding 392 degrees Farenheit

GARLIC ROASTED CANNABIS OIL

YIELDS 7.5 MG OF THC PER TBSP.

2 heads of peeled garlic

1 gram of ground cannabis product

16 ounces high temperature canola oil

Cheesecloth

INSTRUCTIONS

Make small sachet with your ground cannabis product using the cheesecloth.

Place oil in 4-quart pot over low heat.

Add sachet of cannabis and cook on low heat for up to 1 ½–2 hours.

Stir occasionally. Do not allow oil to boil.

Allow oil to cool and then strain using a chinois or layered cheesecloth set into a strainer.

CHILI INFUSED CANNABIS OIL

YIELDS 7.5 MG OF THC PER TBSP.

3 large seeded guajillo chilies

2 large seeded ancho chilies

½ cup arbol chili

1 gram of ground cannabis product

16 ounces high temperature canola oil

Cheesecloth

INSTRUCTIONS

Make small sachet with your ground cannabis product, using the cheesecloth.

Put seeded peppers in large pot. Add sachet and pour in oil.

Cook on low heat for to 2–3 hours.

Stir occasionally. Do not allow oil to boil.

Allow oil to cool and then strain using a chinois or layered cheesecloth set into a strainer.

*For an extended shelf life on oil products, store in a dark bottle and keep in cool dry place or refrigerator

DRESSINGS, JAMS, AND PUREES

BACON JAM

YIELDS 2 CUPS AT 60 MG OF THC PER CUP

1 lb. thick cut bacon

2 large sweet onions (halved and sliced)

½ cup brown sugar

2 Tbsp. maple syrup (reference recipe on next page)

⅓ cup infused strong brew coffee (reference recipe on next page)

1 Tbsp. mustard seeds

1 Tbsp. balsamic vinegar

¼ tsp. cayenne pepper

½ tsp. salt

INSTRUCTIONS

Dice the bacon and add to a large skillet. Cook over medium-high heat, stirring frequently until the bacon is cooked through. Make sure the frying yields chewy bacon versus crispy bacon.

Remove from the skillet and set aside. Pour off most of the bacon drippings, leaving some to cook the onions.

Add the onions to the skillet and then salt. Cook on low heat and stir consistently for 20 minutes or until the onions are nicely caramelized. Add sugar and cook for another 5–7 minutes while stirring. Add the maple syrup, coffee, water, mustard seeds, and bacon.

Cook on medium heat until the mixture is of a jam consistency, stirring every 5 minutes. Remove from heat and stir in the balsamic vinegar.

Cool and refrigerate for up to one week. There will be little spots. Bring to room temperature before serving.

HOMEMADE MAPLE SYRUP

YIELDS 32 SERVINGS AT 7.5 MG PER SERVING

1 cup water

1 cup turbinado sugar

1 cup brown sugar

1 Tbsp. maple flavored extract

1 gram ground cannabis sachet

INSTRUCTIONS

In a saucepan bring cannabis sachet, water, and sugars to a boil over medium-high heat. Reduce heat to medium low and add maple extract. Simmer for 3–5 minutes or until desired richness is achieved.

INFUSED STRONG BREW COFFEE

YIELDS 3 CUPS AT 180 MG OF THC PER CUP

6 cups freshly brewed coffee

3 grams cannabis product

Cheesecloth

Kitchen grade twine

INSTRUCTIONS

Create a sachet of cannabis product using the cheesecloth and kitchen grade twine.

Place coffee in a medium-sized saucepan and bring to a low heat. Add sachet and reduce the coffee by one half to 3 cups.

Strain and cool.

*Besides being used for the bacon jam recipe above, this product can also be used in cakes, bread puddings, milkshakes, cookies, frappes, etc.

** Recipes based on product containing 18% THC

 BUD PAIRING: For this recipe, I used a rare CHOCOLATE DIESEL strain, as it has coffee notes with woodsy undertones. An alternative is Chocolate Thai, which also has a coffee flavor along with notes of spice. Both have euphoric and energetic properties that add an additional boost to infused coffee.

FIG PRESERVES

YIELDS 3 ½ PINT JARS (24 OUNCES TOTAL) AT 4.5 MG PER OUNCE/SERVING

2 lbs. purple figs (stemmed and diced)

3 hefty sprigs of thyme

½ gram of cannabis product

1½ cups sugar

¼ cup fresh lemon juice

½ cup white port wine

3 sterilized half-pint canning jars

Cheesecloth

Kitchen grade cotton twine

INSTRUCTIONS

Create a small sachet of cannabis product using the cheesecloth and kitchen grade twine. Place figs, sachet, and sugar in large saucepan and let stand. Stir occasionally for 15 minutes until sugar is mostly dissolved.

Add the lemon juice, thyme sprigs, and white port and bring to a boil, stirring until the sugar is completely dissolved.

Cook over medium heat for roughly 20 minutes until the figs are soft and the liquid comes to a thick syrupy consistency.

Discard the sprigs of thyme and spoon the jam into 3 half-pint canning jars, leaving a quarter inch of space at the top. Close the jars and let cool to room temperature.

 BUD PAIRING: For this recipe, I've use organic and outdoor grown Girl Scout Cookies. Its sweet yet earthy texture balances well with natural sugars in figs.

* Recipes based on product containing 22% THC

BALSAMIC RASPBERRY PRESERVES

YIELDS 4 CUPS (32 OUNCES) AT 6.25 MG OF THC PER OUNCE/SERVING

4 cups granulated bakers sugar

4 cups raspberries

1 cup of quality balsamic vinegar

1 gram sachet of cannabis product

INSTRUCTIONS

In a small saucepan, bring the balsamic vinegar with the cannabis sachet to a boil on medium to high heat. Once boiling, lower the temperature and cook until the balsamic vinegar reduces to a thick syrup consistency. Tend to it carefully, as it can turn and burn easily. Reduce to about three-quarters to one-half the original volume. Set aside and allow to cool.

Meanwhile, place sugar in an ovenproof pan and warm in a 250°F (120°C) oven for 15 minutes.

Place berries in a large saucepan. Bring to a boil over high heat, mashing the berries as they heat. Boil hard for 1 minute, stirring constantly.

Add warm sugar and boil until mixture forms a gel (approximately 5 minutes). The consistency should be thick and should drip slowly from the back of a spoon. Strain balsamic reduction and add to the raspberry mixture. If needed, cook additionally to resume the proper consistency.

Spoon the jam into sterilized jars leaving ¼ of a space at the top. Process 10 minutes in boiling water deep enough to cover lids by at least 1 inch.

* Recipes based on product containing 22% THC

WATERMELON PRESERVES

YIELDS 6 CUPS AT 360 MG (SERVING SIZE 1 TBSP. AT 3.75 MG PER)

6 cups watermelon rind, diced

4½ cups sugar

Juice of 1 lemon

2 Tbsp. lemon zest

1½ g sachet of cannabis product

INSTRUCTIONS

Peel away the green from the watermelon yet leave bits of the red pulp intact. Dice and place the rinds in a large pot. Add the cannabis product sachet and cover with sugar so that the rind is not visible. Cover the contents and refrigerate overnight.

Place pot on stove and add lemon juice. Bring the mixture to a boil, cooking for 2 hours and until the rind is clear. Remove from heat. Squeeze out the sachet and discard.

Spoon the preserves into sterilized jars. Process 10 minutes in boiling water deep enough to cover lids by at least 1 inch.

* Recipes based on product containing 24% THC

CANNABIS INFUSED BUTTERMILK

YIELDS 1 QUART AT 50 MG OF THC PER CUP

1 quart buttermilk

1 cup water

2 gram sachet of cannabis product

INSTRUCTIONS

In a saucepan, bring the buttermilk and water to a boil. Add the sachet of cannabis and lower the heat. Allow to simmer for 40 minutes. Stir occasionally to ensure that the milk does not scald. Remove from heat and cool; squeeze out sachet and discard.

*Product can also be used for pancakes, biscuits, etc.

** Recipes based on product containing 10% THC

BUD PAIRING: Jamaican Lion pairs well for this recipe. It has flavors of lime with sweet herbal notes on the back palate. I also favor this strain because it is CBD-rich and has mild THC levels.

BUTTERMILK DILL DRESSING

YIELDS 1 CUP AT 25 MG (SERVING SIZE 1 OUNCE AT 6.25 G PER)

½ cup cannabis infused buttermilk (reference recipe)

¾ cup crème fraîche

¼ cup mayonnaise

½ Tbsp. dry mustard

1 large garlic clove (minced)

1 tsp. kosher salt

1 Tbsp. champagne vinegar

¼ tsp. white pepper

4 Tbsp. dill (finely chopped)

INSTRUCTIONS

Add all ingredients, with the exception of the cannabis infused buttermilk, to a bowl and mix thoroughly. Whisk in the buttermilk until it is smooth and creamy.

PEANUT DRESSING

YIELDS 2 ½ CUPS (20 OUNCES) AT 110 MG OF THC (11 MG PER SERVING/2 OUNCES)

½ cup olive oil

1 tsp. sesame oil

1 ½ cups of smooth peanut butter

½ coconut milk

3 Tbsp. soy sauce

6 Tbsp. water

3 Tbsp. lime juice

1 Tbsp. fish sauce

1 Tbsp. fresh ginger (minced)

3 garlic cloves (minced)

1 Thai chili pepper (minced)

1 Tbsp. black sesame seeds

½ gram sachet of cannabis product

INSTRUCTIONS

In a small saucepan, bring coconut milk and water to a boil. Add sachet of cannabis product and bring heat to a low simmer. Cook on low heat for 15 minutes, stirring occasionally. If the mixture thickens, add an additional Tbsp. of water.

Remove from heat and allow it to cool. Squeeze out the sachet and discard.

Add the infused coconut milk to a bowl and whisk in peanut butter, soy sauce, fish sauce, lime juice, Thai chili, ginger, garlic, and sesame seeds.

* Recipes based on product containing 22% THC

RASPBERRY BALSAMIC VINAIGRETTE

YIELDS ¼ CUP AT 12.5 MG OF THC (3.125 MG OF THC PER TBSP.)

⅛ cup balsamic vinegar

⅛ cup quality olive oil

2 Tbsp. balsamic raspberry preserves (reference recipe)

½ onion powder

1 Tbsp. Dijon mustard

¼ tsp. salt

INSTRUCTIONS

Whisk together the olive oil, balsamic vinegar, raspberry preserves, onion powder, Dijon mustard, and salt in a small bowl until smooth.

GINGER PEACH PUREE

YIELDS 2 CUPS AT 220 MG TOTAL (13.75 MG PER 1 OUNCE SERVING)

4 medium-sized peaches (pitted and sliced)

2 Tbsp. ginger (minced)

1 tsp. lemon zest

1 cup sugar

4 cups water

1 gram sachet of cannabis product

INSTRUCTIONS

Add all ingredients with the exception of the lemon zest and cannabis sachet to a large pot. Bring to a high boil and add the cannabis sachet, and then lower temperature. Simmer the mixture on low heat for 1 hour.

Remove from heat, add lemon zest, and cool. Blend the mixture to a fine consistency and press through a chinois.

* Recipes based on product containing 22% THC

VEGETABLES, LEGUMES, FRUITS, AND FUNGUS

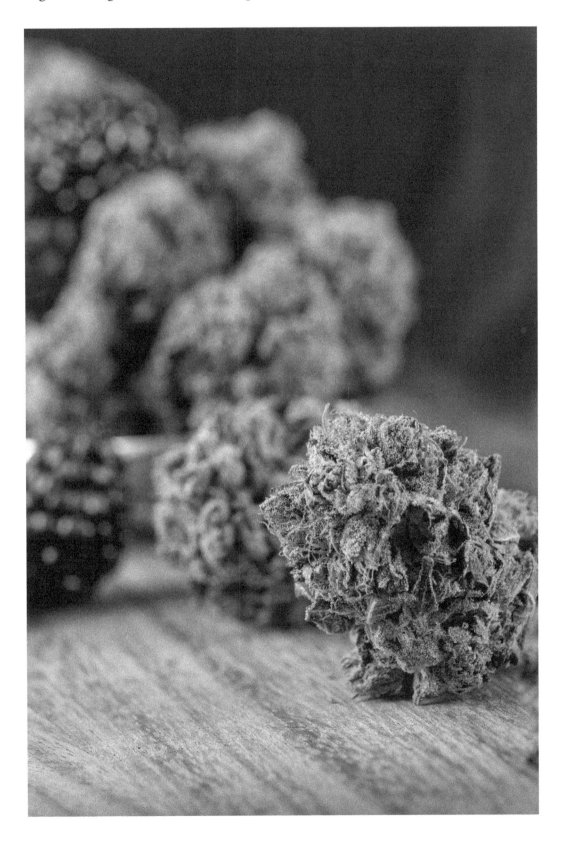

There is a power to the memory of food that verges on the beautiful. It can elicit a smile, a grimace, even a tear. Food memory—better than a time travel rocket— can spin you back decades, to when you sat shoulder-to-shoulder with a dining partner. It can teleport you to the crook of a tree, biting into the ripened flesh of a mango. It can, in a half second, fill your mouth with a stiff mound of cold grits, its grains trapped in spaces between your teeth.

A person can live a lifetime of curiosity based on food memory (remember Proust's Madeleine?) A single bad food memory can be the death of future opportunity. I think of food memory as the culinary Achilles heel. It has the power to deprive us of new experiences, and most of the heels, in my opinion, have to do with vegetables.

How often have you seen a friend cringe at the mention of spinach, beets, or peas? Or heard a mate's nervous voice pleading, "oh, I don't eat..." Predicated on a ghastly occurrence, they've sworn off the possibilities of all ...whatevers! As a professional chef, the very idea makes me moan and challenges me to create something for this person to offer them a renewed and positive experience.

At a time, my particular Achilles heel was the Brussels sprout. Eyes wide open; in memory, I can revisit my mother's old kitchen circa 1986. We owned a pale yellow refrigerator that was often filled with frozen things: bags of succotash, green peas, petrified okra, spinach, and yes, Brussels sprouts. She'd remove a bag and place it atop the counter to allow it to defrost. Hours later, I would sit contemplating the mound of mush, begging to know, "why?"

Even at a young age, I was acutely aware of and curious about the distinct difference between the frozen bags that doubled as ice packs and the sun-ripened fields of vegetables lining the back roads of my mother's hometown of Statesboro, GA. I suppose, however, that having experienced the juxtaposition of the two worlds kept me curious enough to give every food a second, third, or fourth chance. The combination of traveling, living in diverse communities, and always keeping an open mind promised me a new experience with the Brussels sprout.

They were eventually reintroduced to me, cooked to just the appropriate give and resting in a warm bath of butter. Later, in Philadelphia, I learned how to roast them with garlic and polish them with olive oil, pine nuts, and aged balsamic. And in New York, I explored a pan-seared version with a white wine and Dijon sauce. Not only does every negative food memory deserve a second chance, but you, too, deserve a renewed, positive experience.

Most food memories are created in our youth under limited circumstances. With greater resources and a world of thriving diversity, we now have magnificent opportunities to create new food memories. Remember, with a slight hint of Berber spice, a rub of garam masala, or the perfect smoke of Jamaican jerk, your culinary Achilles heel can become a welcomed part of a dining excursion.

BEET PASTA HANKERCHIEFS / ROASTED BEETS & BROWN BUTTER SAUCE

YIELDS 7 SERVINGS AT 5.7 MG THC PER SERVING

BRAISED BEET PASTA

YIELDS 7 1-OUNCE SERVINGS OF DOUGH AT 5 MG OF THC PER

6 ounces Tipo 00 Italian flour

2 ounces all-purpose flour

3 medium egg yolks

1 medium egg

1 large beet (peeled and quartered)

1 cup pomegranate juice

1 ¼ cup water

1 cup balsamic vinegar

¾ tsp. cannabis oil

½ Tbsp. water

INSTRUCTIONS

Braised Beet Puree:

Place wine, water, and balsamic vinegar into saucepan. Add the peeled and quartered beet. Bring to boil. Lower the temperature to medium heat. Cook for 5 minutes. Bring temperature to low heat. Cook until the beet is fork-tender.

Reduce remaining liquid until it is a light syrup consistency. Add beets and light syrup to blender and puree until smooth.

Beet Pasta:

Sift Tipo and all-purpose flour. Add into mixer. Turn mixer on low, and add egg yolks one at a time. Then add the full egg. Mix on low, and slowly add the beet puree and cannabis oil. Add water.

Mix until ball forms. Add additional all-purpose flour in small amounts if needed. Knead the dough on a lightly floured surface. Cover in plastic wrap and refrigerate for at least 30 minutes.

Portion the dough into 1-ounce balls. Roll out using a pasta machine.

PASTA FILLING

YIELDS 7 1-OUNCE SERVINGS AT .35 MG PER

4 ounces ricotta cheese (strained)

2½ ounces soft goat cheese

½ ounce grated pecorino cheese

1 tsp. roasted garlic infused oil

1 shallot (minced)

1 garlic clove (minced)

½ cup of beet greens (cleaned and stemmed)

1 tsp. chopped tarragon

Pinch of salt

Sauté beet greens, garlic, and shallots in ½ tsp. of roasted garlic infused oil (reserve the second ½ tsp.). Cook until tender.

Cool and chop fine.

In a bowl, mix the beet greens, ½ tsp. infused roasted garlic oil, cheeses, and chopped tarragon. Set aside for plating.

ROASTED BEETS

¼ lb. Red beets (peeled and halved)

¼ Golden beets (peeled and halved)

¼ cup olive oil

1 tsp. kosher salt

INSTRUCTIONS

Coat the beets in olive oil and salt. Add to a baking dish, and roast for 35–40 minutes at 400 degrees. Turn beets as necessary. Cool, quarter, toss in olive oil, and set aside for plating.

BROWN BUTTER SAUCE

YIELDS 7 1-OUNCE SERVINGS AT .35 MG PER

½ lb. butter clarified butter

¼ Tbsp. clean cannabis butter

6 ounces crème fraîche

1 garlic cloves (minced)

¼ tsp. chopped parsley

¼ chopped tarragon

INSTRUCTIONS

Melt clean cannabis butter and clarified butter in a skillet. Stirring frequently, add chopped tarragon and cook until butter begins to brown. Add minced garlic and cook until soft. Whisk in crème fraîche, and then add the chopped parsley.

TO PLATE:

Center a 1-ounce quenelle of the cheese mixture onto plate. Cover with cooked pasta sheets. Add roasted beet quarters. Spoon hot brown butter sauce over the pasta. Garnish with roasted pistachios or walnuts.

ROASTED & CHARRED TOMATO SALAD WITH ROMESCO SAUCE

YIELDS 4 SERVINGS AT 15.8 MG PER SERVING

12 grape sized heirloom tomatoes

2 medium heirloom tomatoes (sliced into eighths each)

2 Tbsp. micro basil (or chiffonade of basil)

1 cup fava beans (blanched)

4 tsp. fried capers

4 cloves black garlic

2 tsp. roasted pine nuts or hazel nuts

4 ounces burrata cheese

1 Tbsp. chili infused cannabis oil

Kosher salt

1 cup romesco sauce (reference recipe)

INSTRUCTIONS

Toss sliced tomatoes in chili oil and pinch of kosher salt. Roast on a sheet pan for 10 minutes at 350 degrees. Allow to cool. Sauté fava beans in a small skillet at a low temperature until cooked through. Set aside for plating. Use a kitchen torch to char grape sized heirloom tomatoes

TO PLATE:

Per plate, add ¼ cup of room temperature Romesco Sauce. Mount 1 ounce of Burrata cheese. Add 4 slices of roasted heirloom tomatoes and 3 charred tomatoes per plate. Add ¼ cup fava beans, 1 tsp. of fried capers, 1 sliced clove of black garlic and ½

tsp. of pine nuts. Garnish with micro basil.

ROMESCO SAUCE

YIELDS 2 ½ CUPS AT ¼ MG PER CUP SERVING

1 red bell pepper

4 medium-size ripe tomatoes (¾–1 lb. total), cored

1 head garlic, sliced in half crosswise

2 tsp. cannabis oil

4 tsp. plus⅓ cup extra virgin olive oil

½ cup blanched almonds

1 dried ancho chili (cored and seeded) flat

1 tsp. salt

2 Tbsp. sherry vinegar

2 Tbsp. red wine blend

½ cup homemade croutons 5 mg (reference recipe)

INSTRUCTIONS

Put the tomatoes, one half of the garlic head, and red bell pepper in a baking pan. Drizzle with a Tbsp. of olive oil, and roast in a 375-degree oven until caramelization develops (about an hour). Be careful not to burn.

Toast the almonds in a small sauté pan on medium heat, using about 1 Tbsp. of olive oil. Keep the pan in a continuous motion so that the almonds do not burn. Cool, and then add the nuts to a food processor along with 1 Tbsp. of garlic.

Sear the ancho chili in the same sauté pan on high heat for about 15 seconds per side. Reconstitute the chili in a cup of hot water until soft. Drain, and then add it to the food processor with the almonds and garlic.

Pulse the ingredients roughly.

Once the tomatoes, red pepper and garlic are caramelized, allow them to cool. Remove the skins from the tomatoes and squeeze the garlic from the pulp. Add all to the food processor. Blend while adding the infused oil and remaining oil in a slow steam. Add the vinegar, blend, and taste. The result should be slightly tangy with a thick yet smooth consistency. Add wine and bread crumbs. Continue to blend. If needed, add additional red wine or small increments of water (for a milder taste).

HOUSE-MADE CROUTONS

YIELDS 3 CUPS CROUTONS AT 5 MG PER ½ CUP

½ lb. French or artisan style bread

12 tsp. roasted garlic infused cannabis oil

⅛ tsp. garlic powder

⅛ tsp. salt (or to taste)

INSTRUCTIONS

Heat the oven to 375°F. Dice bread into medium-sized cubes. Add to a bowl and toss with oil or butter. Put croutons onto a baking sheet in a single layer. Bake for 5 minutes. Toss croutons. Bake an additional 5 minutes. Croutons may cook longer to a browner tone if desired and depending on the coarseness of the bread.

PAN-SEARED OKRA W/ KALAMATA OLIVES, PECANS & SUNDRIED TOMATO

YIELDS 4 SERVINGS AT 7.75 MG OF THC PER SERVING

2 cups okra (sliced in half lengthwise)

1 cup Kalamata olives

1 cup sundried tomatoes

4 Tbsp. roasted pecan pieces

1 tsp. garlic powder

⅛ tsp. cumin

1 Tbsp. garlic roasted infused oil

½ tsp. cannabis oil

2 Tbsp. olive oil

Kosher salt (to taste)

Pinch of light brown sugar

INSTRUCTIONS

Add garlic, olive, and cannabis oil to large skillet. Place on medium heat until it arrives at a smoke point. Add okra to the skillet. Cook until okra develops a char on the inner sides. Add the cumin, garlic powder, and brown sugar. Add sundried tomatoes and cook for an additional 2 minutes. Add Kalamata olives. Garnish with roasted pecans.

CUCUMBER WATERMELON SALAD & INFUSED POMEGRANATE REDUCTION

YIELDS 6 SERVINGS AT 7.5 MG OF THC PER SERVING

6 2x4 inch watermelon rectangles

6 fennel stems

Kosher salt

12 2x4 slices of cucumber

6–8 tsp. of feta cheese

2 cups of pomegranate juice

1 cup balsamic vinegar

1 cup of pistachios (crushed)

1 Tbsp. red pepper corn (crushed)

Quarter gram sachet of cannabis material

Place 3 watermelon rectangles in a plastic bag along with a few pinches of salt and pink ½ tsp. of pink pepper corns. Vacuum seal the bag. Repeat and refrigerate overnight.

In a small saucepan, bring the balsamic vinegar and pomegranate juice to a boil over high heat. Add the cannabis product sachet; cook for 2 minutes then lower the temperature to a simmer. Reduce mixture by ½ (1½ cups). Remove from heat, discard sachet, and allow it to cool.

Remove watermelon rectangles and pat dry. Plate it by layering a few pearls of the pomegranate reduction onto the top of the watermelon rectangle. Follow it up with 2 slices of cucumber, a thin layer of feta cheese, a thin layer of pistachios, and finish with a sprinkling of finely crushed pink peppercorn. Add reduction to finished plate.

*For plating, pour the mixture into a small squeeze bottle

**Recipe based on product containing 18% THC

 BUD PAIRING: I created this salad based on a client's medical diagnoses. I used a few southern favorites that paired well with the citrus flavor of the Orange Bud hybrid strain. It also has a propensity to be slightly pungent which balances perfectly with the earthy flavors of the pomegranate and balsamic reduction.

GARLIC GREENS & CORN BREAD CROUTONS

YIELDS 4 SERVINGS AT 15 MG OF THC PER SERVING

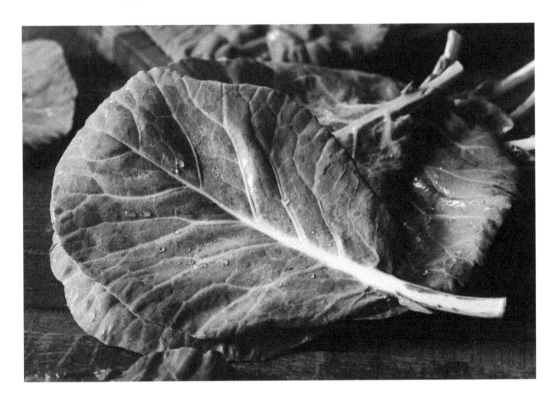

GARLIC GREENS

YIELDS 4 SERVINGS AT 8 MG OF THC PER TBSP.

8 cups collard greens (cleaned and chopped into strips)

1 bottle of white wine

6 cups water

1¾ tsp. butter

¼ tsp. clean cannabis butter

5 cloves garlic (minced)

2 Tbsp. chili infused cannabis oil

Kosher salt to taste

INSTRUCTIONS

In a stockpot, combine the bottle of wine and water and bring to a boil. Allow the combination to reduce slightly. Add chopped collard greens to the pot and blanch. Once the greens are bright in color and softened, remove them from the water and put in an ice bath to stop the cooking process. Once cool, strain and pat dry.

Heat the butter and oil at a medium-high temperature in a skillet. Add minced garlic. Lower temperature and cook until the garlic is translucent, being careful not to let it burn. Add chopped collard greens and sauté. Cook until warmed through. Serve with Cornbread croutons.

CORN BREAD CROUTONS

YIELDS 10 SERVINGS AT 7 MG THC PER SERVING

17 tsp. butter

1 tsp. clean cannabis butter

1 cup cornmeal

¾ cup all-purpose flour

1 Tbsp. sugar

2 large jalapeños (seeded and diced)

2 tsp. paprika

1 ½ tsp. Cajun seasoning

1 tsp. garlic powder

1 ½ tsp. baking powder

½ tsp. baking soda

¼ tsp. salt

2 large eggs

1 ½ cups milk

2 Tbsp. olive oil

INSTRUCTIONS

Prepare an 8-inch baking dish by brushing it with oil. Preheat oven at 425 degrees.

In a large bowl, combine cornmeal, sugar, flour, baking soda, baking powder, paprika, Cajun seasoning, salt, and jalapeno. In a separate bowl, combine cooled melted butter, eggs, and milk.

Combine both mixtures and fold together thoroughly. Pour the batter into a baking dish and cook until golden brown.

Remove from the oven and cool. Turn out the cornbread cut into crouton-sized squares. You can also do a rustic tare. Just assure that the size of the croutons is proportionate.

Place croutons on a baking sheet and drizzle with roasted garlic infused oil. Cook on low temperature until outside of croutons is golden and crusty.

FRENCH ONION SOUP

YIELDS 7 SERVINGS AT 30 MG THC PER SERVING

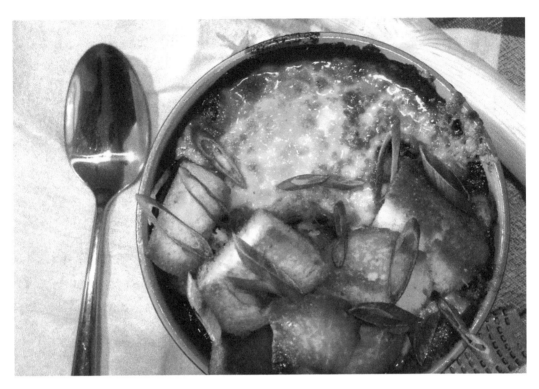

2 lbs. yellow onions (sliced thin)

1 Tbsp. cooking oil

1Tbsp. butter

1 Tbsp. clean cannabis butter

½tsp. sugar

1 tsp. salt

3 Tbsp. flour

6 cups veal stock

1 cup Blue Moon (or other Belgium Ale)

½ cup sherry

1 Tbsp. rosemary (chopped fine)

1 Tbsp. shallots (minced)

1 bay leaf

½ tsp. ground sage

Kosher salt to taste

12 ounces Gruyère cheese (grated)

4 ounces Fontina cheese (grated)

2 ounces Colby Jack cheese (grated)

½ raw yellow onion

2–3 Tbsp. cognac

House-made croutons (reference recipe)

4 Tbsp. olive oil (for drizzling)

INSTRUCTIONS

Place heavy bottom stockpot over medium-low heat. Add 1 Tbsp. cooking oil, 1 Tbsp. butter, and 1 Tbsp. cannabis butter to pot. Add sliced onions and stir until they are evenly coated with the oil. Cover and cook for about 20 minutes until they are very tender and translucent.

To brown or caramelize the onions, turn heat under pot to medium or medium-high heat. Add 1/2 tsp. sugar and 1 tsp. salt and continue to cook uncovered, stirring frequently until the onions have browned and reduced significantly.

Once caramelized, reduce heat to medium-low and add 3 Tbsp. flour to the onions. Brown the flour for about 2–3 minutes, trying not to scorch it. (If the flour does not form a thick paste, add a bit more butter here.) Stir in about 1 cup of warm stock, scraping the bottom of the pan to get up all of the cooked-on bits. Add the rest of the stock, beer, sherry, sage, and bay leaf to the soup. Simmer for 30 minutes.

Transfer to 7 individual small oven safe bowls. At this point you can add the 2–3 Tbsp. cognac and grate the half raw onion into the soup. Add a few ounces of the Gruyère cheese directly into the soup and stir. Place the croutons in a single layer on top of the soup. Sprinkle the rest of the cheese in a thick layer on top of the bread, making sure to cover the edges of the toast to prevent burning. Drizzle with a little oil or melted butter.

Place in a 350-degree oven for about 30 minutes. Turn on broiler and brown cheese well at the end.

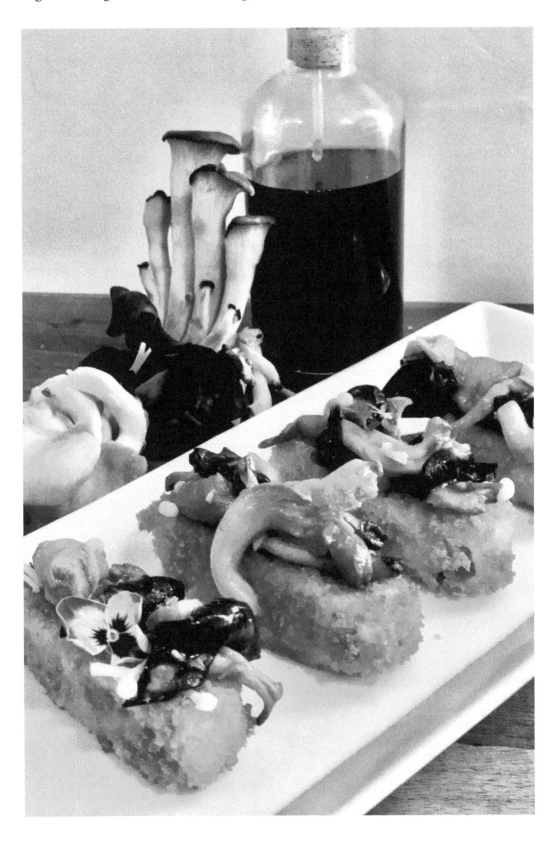

CRISPY POLENTA W/ MUSHROOM RAGOUT

YIELDS 8 SERVINGS AT 14.6 MG PER SERVING

MUSHROOM RAGOUT

YIELDS 8 SERVINGS AT 1.875 MG PER SERVING

2 lbs. mixed fresh wild mushrooms

2 Tbsp. roasted garlic and chive cannabis butter

2 shallots (chopped fine)

Pinch of cayenne pepper

1½ cups vegetable stock

6 Tbsp. vegetable demi-glace

½ cup sour cream

4 sprigs fresh thyme

Kosher salt

⅛ tsp. white pepper

INSTRUCTIONS

Trim and slice mushrooms. In a large skillet, melt the butter over medium heat adding finely chopped shallots. Stir occasionally and cook until tender.

Add mushrooms. Cook until the mushroom liquids are released. Add the vegetable stock and cook for an additional 5 minutes. Then add the vegetable demi-glace, cream, cayenne, and white pepper. Cook for an additional 5 minutes. Finish with fresh thyme.

CRISPY POLENTA

YIELDS 8 SERVINGS AT 12.75 MG PER SERVING

1 ¾ cup cornmeal

3 cups water

1 cup cream

1 ½ tsp. clean cannabis butter (reference recipe)

½ cup sharp white cheddar

½ cup triple cream Brie (or desired cheese)

Kosher salt to taste

4 cups panko breadcrumbs

2 eggs

1 ½ cups all-purpose flour

1 quart canola oil

INSTRUCTIONS

Lightly brush an 8x8 baking dish with cannabis oil. Set aside.

Salt 2 cups of water and 1 cup cream, and bring to a boil in a medium-sized stockpot. Sprinkle in cornmeal while whisking. Lower the temperature on saucepan. Add additional water as needed. Cornmeal should remain at the consistency of creamy grits. Whisk constantly and cook for about 30 minutes.

Add cannabis butter, white cheddar, and Brie. Whisk until it is smooth and creamy. Pour creamy mixture into oiled 8x8 baking dish. Cool for 10 minutes. Lay plastic wrap directly onto polenta, and allow it to set up overnight in refrigerator.

After it has set, remove polenta and unmold on a sizeable cutting board. Cut into 8 logs (approximately 4x2)

Pour canola oil into a stockpot, and bring to a temperature of 350 degrees

Add ¼ cup of water to the 2 eggs and mix thoroughly. Create 2 separate bowls of all-purpose flour and panko breadcrumbs.

Dip logs first into flour, then egg bath, and then panko breadcrumbs. Deep-fry them (2–3 at a time) until golden brown.

*Garnish with thinly sliced button mushrooms, butter poached peas, and micro greens

*Adding too many logs to the hot oil will lower the temperature, thus making it more challenging to get an even cook. It could also cause the polenta logs to be weighed down with oil.

CORN CUSTARD W/ CRAB & FENNEL SALAD

YIELDS 6 SERVINGS AT 20 MG OF THC PER SERVING

1 Tbsp. butter

2 cups roasted corn (roasted and cut from the cob)

1½ cups corn (roasted and pan-fried for plating)

1½ cups heavy whipping cream

1 tsp. kosher salt

⅛ tsp. smoked paprika

¼ Thai chili pepper (minced)

½ cup cold milk

3 large egg yolks

2 eggs

½ gram sachet of cannabis material

INSTRUCTIONS

Butter 6 6-ounce ceramic ramekins. Place into a 2-inch deep baking dish.

Place cream and cannabis material sachet into saucepan. Bring to a low heat, and cook for 20 minutes. Add 2 cups of roasted corn and minced chili pepper. Cook for another 10 minutes on low heat. Stir in salt and smoked paprika. Remove from heat, and then stir in the milk. Squeeze out the sachet and discard.

Blend corn mixture until smooth. Temper a quarter cup of the hot mixture into a bowl of well-whisked egg yolks and eggs. Whisk until smooth. Slowly add the additional corn mixture until all is well combined. Transfer corn mixture to a blender, and pulse several times to get the mixture moving. Blend on high speed until smooth and creamy.

Divide the mixture equally into the 6 ramekins. Carefully pour water into the baking dish to the halfway point of the ramekins. Bake in a 325-degree preheated oven for about 30 minutes. Allow custards to cool for about 5 minutes before serving.

To unmold, insert a knife between the custard and the ramekin, go around the edge with the knife to loosen, and turn over onto a plate to unmold into prepared cornhusk.

CRAB & FENNEL SALAD

YIELDS 6 SERVINGS AT 20 MG OF THC PER SERVING

3 ounces jumbo lump crab

½ ounce fennel (sliced thin)

½ tsp. apple cider vinegar

1 tsp. olive oil (may be substituted with infused chili oil for enhanced version)

1Tbsp. Thyme (chopped)

Kosher salt to taste

Pinch of granulated sugar

INSTRUCTIONS

Whisk together vinegar and oil. Add sugar, salt, and thyme. Stir.

Fold in fennel. Move around for a minute or so until the fennel gives and softens. Gently fold in crab, being careful not to break up the lump meat.

Serve on top of corn custard with pan-fried corn.

ROASTED PEAR SALAD

YIELDS 8 MG OF THC PER TBSP

3 bartlett pears (halved and cored)

3 cups spring mix

½ cup parsley

½ cup fennel (thinly sliced)

½ cup mint (roughly chopped)

2 tsp. thyme

2 Tbsp. olive oil

1 Tbsp. raw sugar

Infused raspberry dressing (reference recipe)

6 Tbsp. blue cheese

Pinch of Salt

INSTRUCTIONS

Toss pears in olive oil and sugar. Roast on a sheet pan at 450 degrees until golden. Remove from the oven and cool.

In a bowl, blend mixed greens, mint, parsley, fennel, and thyme, and salt to taste. Serve with raspberry dressing and blue cheese.

Optional: Garnish with raspberries, blueberries, and/or toasted walnuts.

CHICKEN FRIED PORTABELLA WITH MUSHROOM BORDELAISE & NEW POTATO SALAD

YIELDS 4 SERVINGS AT 10.4 MG OF THC PER SERVING

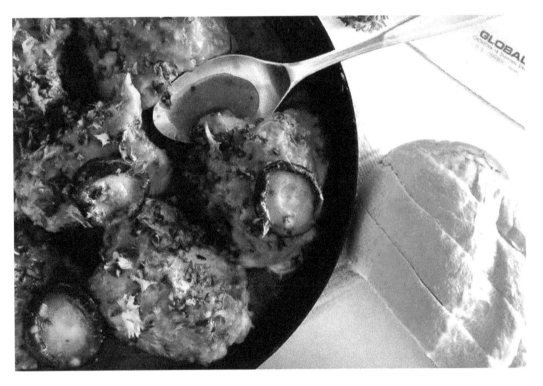

4 large portabella mushrooms

8 sprigs of thyme

8 garlic cloves

4 tsp. whole peppercorns

4 bay leaves

2 cups vegetable stock

3 cups garbanzo flour (all-purpose flour can be substituted)

3 Tbsp. Cajun seasoning

1 Tbsp. paprika

½ Tbsp. smoked paprika

2 Tbsp. garlic powder

1½ tsp. cayenne pepper

1 tsp. cumin

1½ Tbsp. kosher salt

3 large eggs

1 quart canola oil

2 cups potato salad

2 cups mushroom bordelaise (reference recipe)

8 Tbsp. (1 stick) of unsalted butter (room temperature)

1 tsp. of clean cannabis butter (room temperature; reference recipe)

1 head of roasted garlic (reference recipe)

2½ Tbsp. of chives (blanched and chopped)

Pinch of salt

Sealable plastic bag

Plastic wrap

INSTRUCTIONS

Place stemmed portabella in a vacuum seal bag. Add a quarter cup vegetable stock, 2 sprigs of thyme, 2 garlic cloves, 1 bay leaf, and 1 tsp. of peppercorn to each bag. Seal and refrigerate, allowing the mushrooms to marinate overnight.

Bring a large stockpot of water to a roaring boil. Insert the sealed mushrooms, and adjust temperature to low heat. Cook for 3–7 minutes, depending on the thickness of your portabellas. The end result should be soft on the outside, yet left with a slightly firm texture in the center. Remove from water and place in an ice bath to cool.

Add the quart of canola oil to a medium-sized stockpot, and bring to 350 degrees.

In a bowl, combine flour, Cajun seasoning, paprika, smoked paprika, garlic powder, cayenne pepper, cumin, and kosher salt. In separate bowl, thoroughly mix the eggs with a quarter cup of water.

Remove the portabellas from the packaging and pat dry. Coat in flour, dredge in egg mixture, then coat a second time in seasoned flour. Repeat for each of the 4 servings. Deep fry until golden brown.

Drain on paper towel, cut in half, and serve with a quarter cup of bordelaise and a quarter cup of potato salad (optional).

*If you don't have a vacuum sealer, use individual storage bags. Push all of the air out of the bag before sealing.

**The portabella marinade can be reused as marinade, sauce reduction, etc.

MUSHROOM BORDELAISE

YIELDS 4 SERVINGS AT 9.6 MG OF THC

1 cup mushroom stock (reference recipe)

2 Tbsp. shallots (minced)

⅓ cup red wine

1 Tbsp. Worcestershire sauce

½ tsp. rosemary

½ tsp. thyme

8 ½ tsp. butter

½ tsp.

1 bay leaf

1 ½ tsp. black peppercorn

1 tsp. garlic (minced)

½ cup of porcini powder (can substitute 2 cups of fresh mushrooms)

1 Tbsp. cornstarch

2 Tbsp. water

INSTRUCTIONS

Melt 1 Tbsp. of butter in a skillet over medium heat. Stir in the garlic and shallot, and cook until softened. Add remaining butter, melt, then stir in porcini powder. Cook and stir constantly for about 5 minutes.

Add thyme and rosemary, and cook until fragrance is released. Add the bay leaf, peppercorns, mushroom stock, Worcestershire sauce, and wine, and simmer over medium-high heat. Cook for about 20 minutes to allow sauce to reduce.

Dissolve the cornstarch in cold water; 93 whisk the mixture into the sauce thoroughly to thicken. Strain the sauce using a fine mesh sieve.

VEGETABLE STOCK

YIELDS 2 QUARTS (64 CUPS) AT 1.7 MG OF THC PER 1 CUP

2 large onions (quartered)

2 leeks (chopped)

5 celery stalks (chopped)

2 large carrot (peeled and chopped)

1 Tbsp. olive oil

5 ounces crimini mushrooms

2 bay leaves

1 sprig rosemary

4 sprigs of thyme

2 1½ cups white port wine

1 head of garlic (halved)

1 fennel bulb (chopped)

1 tsp. whole black peppercorns

1 Tbsp. tomato paste

½ gram sachet of cannabis product

INSTRUCTIONS

Heat the oil in a large stockpot over medium-high heat. Add all ingredients except sachet, tomato paste, wine, and water. Cook until the vegetables begin to soften.

Add the tomato paste and cook until it begins to slightly caramelize (darken). Deglaze the vegetables with the port wine. Cook until the wine reduces. Add 4 quarts of cold water, bring to a boil, then reduce to a low simmer until the stock is reduced by half, 1–1½ hours.

Strain, pressing to release all of the liquids. Cool in an ice bath. Freeze and use as needed.

DO AHEAD: Stock can be made 3 days ahead. Let cool completely, then cover and chill, or freeze for up to 3 months.

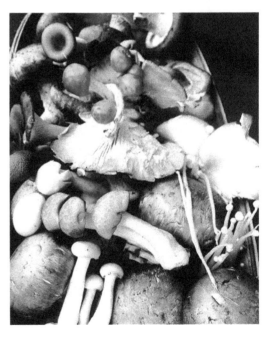

MUSHROOM STOCK

YIELDS 2 QUARTS (64 CUPS) AT 3.43 MG OF THC PER 1 CUP

1 large yellow onion (quartered)

2 cups mushroom stems

2 ounces dried shiitake mushrooms

1 cup fresh assorted mushroom tops

1 leek (chopped)

1 head of garlic (halved)

1 bay leaf

2 celery stalks

1 tsp. peppercorns

1 gram sachet of cannabis material

2 Tbsp. roasted garlic cannabis oil (reference recipe)

1½ cups dry white wine

4 quarts of water

INSTRUCTIONS

Heat roasted garlic infused oil in a stockpot. Add onions, chopped celery, peppercorns, leek, and bay leaf. Cook until onion is translucent. Add head of garlic, and cook for another 4 minutes. Increase the heat, and add mushroom stems, shitake mushrooms, and assorted mushroom tops. Cook another 3 minutes. Deglaze with white wine, and lower the heat. Allow the wine to reduce. Add 4 quarts of cold water, bring to a boil, then reduce to a low simmer until the stock is reduced by half. Strain, pressing out as much liquid as possible.

Cool in an ice bath. Freeze and use as needed.

*Recipes based on product containing 22% THC

BUD PAIRING: Girl Scout Cookies is a strain that I use regularly for its earthy texture. Its subtle air of sweetness balances well will with a variety of recipes. This hybrid strain works seamlessly with mushroom stock. My purveyor offers an organic outdoor grown version with levels of THC at **22%**.

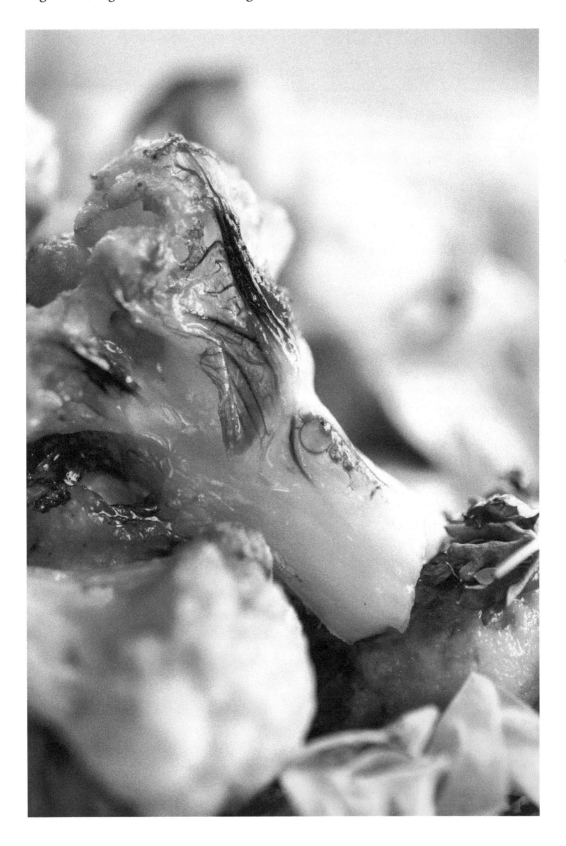

BROCCOLI W/ ROASTED CAULIFLOWER, FRIED SCALLIONS

YIELDS 6 SERVINGS AT 18.8 MG PER SERVING

2 Tbsp. butter

1 large onion (chopped)

1 stalk celery (chopped)

3 cups vegetable broth

8 cups broccoli florets

*½ Tbsp. clean cannabis butter
(reference recipe)*

½ Tbsp. butter

1 Tbsp. flour

*1 avocado
(peeled and tossed in fresh lemon juice)*

1½ cups cream

½ cup milk

2 cups cauliflower florets

*1 Tbsp. roasted garlic cannabis oil
(reference recipe)*

¼ tsp. kosher salt

¼ tsp. cilantro

INSTRUCTIONS

Toss cauliflower in roasted garlic infused oil with ¼ tsp. salt. Place on a roasting pan, and cook at 350 degrees for 10–15 minutes or until golden and tender. Cool and toss with cilantro. Plate in the center of the bowl before ladling in broccoli soup.

Melt 2 Tbsp. butter in a medium-sized stockpot. Add onion and sauté until caramelized (30 minutes) stirring frequently. Add celery and cook until tender. Incorporate an additional and small amount of butter or oil if needed. Add the broccoli and the vegetable broth. Cover and simmer for 10 minutes.

Pour some of the mixture into blender to the halfway mark. Blend until smooth. Continue in batches, adding the avocado to the final batch. Pour into a clean stockpot.

In a separate saucepan, melt one half Tbsp. of clean cannabis butter and one half Tbsp. of butter. Add one half Tbsp. of flour. Stir until slightly golden, and then whisk in cream and milk. Add mixture to soup. Allow to simmer while plating cauliflower. Ladle into bowls. Garnish with fried shallots and steamed English.

 BUD PAIRING: The Pandora's Box strain came to me through a colleague who also grows organically. I paired it with this recipe and found its uplifting properties to work well. The flavor profile of this sativa is amazing with this broccoli soup with its full-bodied peppery flavors.

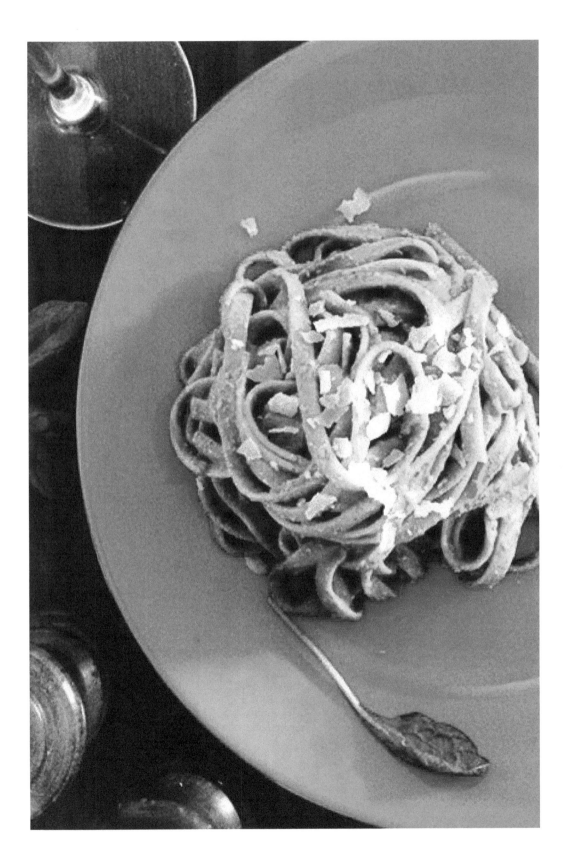

PASTAS AND BREADS

PASTA DOUGH

YIELDS 7 1-OUNCE SERVINGS OF DOUGH AT 5 MG PER SERVING

6 ounces Tipo 00 Italian flour

2 ounces all-purpose flour

3 medium egg yolks

1 medium egg

1¼ cup water

1 cup balsamic vinegar

¼ tsp. cannabis oil (reference recipe)

½ Tbsp. water

INSTRUCTIONS

Sift Tipo and all-purpose flour. Add into mixer. Turn mixer on low and add egg yolks one at a time. Then add the full egg. Mix on low and slowly add the cannabis oil.

Add water.

Mix until ball forms. Add additional all-purpose flour in small amounts if needed. Knead the dough on lightly floured surface. Cover in plastic wrap and refrigerate for at least 30 minutes.

Portion the dough into 1-ounce balls. Roll out using a pasta machine.

SPAGHETTI & MEAT SAUCE

YIELDS 10 SERVINGS AT 14.1 MG PER SERVING

12 fresh tomatoes (peeled, chopped, and blended in a food processor)

4 cloves of garlic

4 Tbsp. micro basil (or chiffonade of basil)

2 tsp. fresh cracked black pepper

1 Tbsp. of cannabis oil (reference recipe)

3 Tbsp. olive oil

1 lb. ground beef

1 lb. spicy Italian sausage

INSTRUCTIONS

Heat 2 Tbsp. olive oil. Add ground beef, spicy Italian sausage, and garlic powder. Cook thoroughly, drain, and set aside.

Tomato Sauce: Peel the skins off of the tomatoes. I recommend that you score the tomatoes first and then blanch them for 1 minute and then place them in cold water. Once they have cooled, the skins should peel off easily. Chop the tomatoes and place them in a blender; control consistency by how long you blend. Shorter blend cycle will yield chunkier sauce; longer blend cycle will yield smoother sauce.

Heat the cannabis oil and olive oil in a large pot (5 quarts or bigger) over medium heat and add chopped garlic, making sure not to burn the garlic. Add tomatoes,

black pepper, basil, sugar, and meat. Stir often. Bring to a low boil. Lower heat and let simmer 2–3 hours, making sure to stir often. For the first half of simmer, do so with the pot uncovered. Cover.

 BUD PAIRING: The strain Sage is a favorite, if you can find it, to use with Italian cuisine. I find that this bud really complements the flavors of the meat and adds a robust and slightly earthy and spicy tone to the sauce. Although it doesn't have the highest THC level (20%), it does have a long lasting effect, which is great for pain management.

STUFFED RAVIOLI

YIELDS 4 SERVINGS AT 8.75 MG PER SERVING

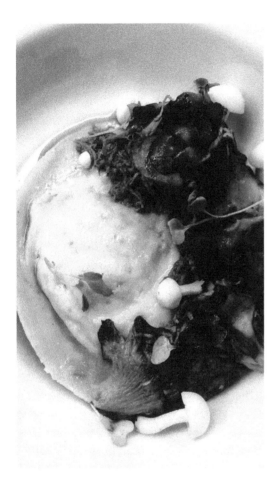

8 ounces ricotta cheese

1 cup freshly grated parmesan cheese

3 tsp. thyme

1 tsp. mint

1 clove garlic

¼ tsp. kosher salt

¼ tsp. white pepper

Nutmeg (to taste)

1 Tbsp. chili infused cannabis oil (reference recipe)

Kosher Salt

1 large egg (lightly beaten)

Pasta dough (reference recipe)

INSTRUCTIONS

Refer to pasta instructions for dough.

Mix all ingredients together well, and fill pasta. Bring a large pot of salted water to a boil. Add ravioli and stir to ensure they separate. Cook uncovered on a gentle boil until the pasta is just tender (2–3 minutes). Drain and serve.

MAC & CHEESE SPHERES

YIELDS 6 SERVINGS AT 15.8 MG PER SERVING

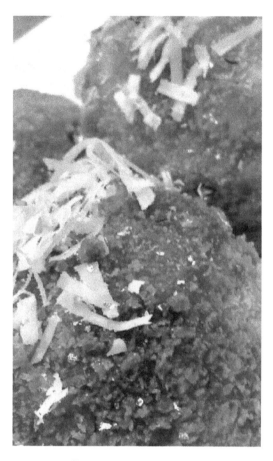

2 Tbsp shallot (diced fine)

2 cups panko

2 eggs

1 cup flour

4 cups oil

INSTRUCTIONS

Bring a pot of water to boil; add salt to water. Cook pasta aldente. Drain and set aside

In another large pot, melt the butter over low heat. Add shallots and cook until softened. Then add thyme and garlic. Cook on medium low heat for another minute. Add flour and stir over medium heat until the mixture is light blonde (1-2 minutes). Add the milk and heavy cream. Whisk to remove any lumps; add the salt and pepper. Cook over medium high heat until the sauce thickens and starts to bubble (6 minutes). Stir in cheese and whisk until smooth and melted. Turn off the heat. Add drained pasta to sauce and mix well.

1 ½ cups elbow macaroni

2 tbsp butter

1 tbsp clean cannabis butter (reference recipe)

3 tbsp all-purpose flour

1 cup milk

1 cup heavy cream

1 cup fontina

½ cup mozzarella,

½ cup gorgonzola

1 Tbsp garlic (minced)

2 Tbsp thyme

Pour mixture into an 8x8 inch pan and allow to cool over night. Fold out onto a clean surface and portion into six squares. Using gloved hands, roll each square into a sphere. Roll the spheres in flour, dusting off any excess, dredge floured spheres in mixture of two beaten eggs and ¼ cup of water. Next press sphere in panko bread crumbs. Deep fry in oil at 340 degrees until golden.

ROSEMARY & WHITE CHEDDAR BISCUITS

YIELDS 12 SERVINGS AT 17.6 MG PER SERVING

1¼ cup bread flour

1¼ cup pastry flour

13 Tbsp. butter

1 Tbsp. clean cannabis butter (reference recipe)

1¼ Tbsp. baking powder

2 Tbsp. sugar

13 ounces milk

2½ tsp. salt

8 ounces white cheddar cheese

¼ cup rosemary

BUD PAIRING: They say what happens in Vegas stays in Vegas, unfortunately that must be the case with this strain. Chloe has a sweet and honey tone that is perfect for a biscuit made with the sharp bite of cheddar. This strain is good for those who suffer from loss of appetite, but too much and you'll find yourself asleep.

INSTRUCTIONS

Sift dry ingredients into a bowl. Break up the butter into the dry ingredients. Mix in mixing bowl until it resembles coarse cornmeal. Add liquid ingredients. Mix liquid ingredients with dry and combine. Knead lightly.

Roll out the dough onto floured surface. Use round or square cookie cutter to portion out 12 servings. Place each biscuit on cooking sheet. Bake at 375 degrees until biscuits are slightly golden.

SAVORY CRACKERS

YIELDS 30 SERVINGS AT 7.06 MG PER SERVING

7 Tbsp. butter

1 Tbsp. clean cannabis butter (reference recipe)

3 ounces grated parmesan

1¼ cups all-purpose flour

¼ tsp. kosher salt

1 tsp. chopped fresh thyme

½ tsp. fresh ground pepper

INSTRUCTIONS

Place butter in a mixer and mix until creamy. Add parmesan, flour, salt, thyme, and pepper. Place dough on lightly floured surface, and roll into 13-inch log. Place the log in plastic wrap and place in the freezer for 30 minutes to harden.

Preheat oven to 350 degrees.

Cut log into half-inch slices. Place on baking sheet, and cook for 22 minutes.

CORN MUFFINS WITH CRISPY BACON AND BACON DRIPPINGS

YIELDS 12 SERVINGS AT 17.6 MG PER SERVING

3 cups all-purpose flour

1 cup sugar

1 cup cornmeal

2 Tbsp. baking powder

1½ tsp. salt

1½ cups whole milk

15 Tbsp. butter (melted and cooled)

1 Tbsp. clean cannabis butter (melted and cooled; reference recipe)

2 large eggs

4 strips cooked bacon (diced)

½ cup corn

INSTRUCTIONS

Preheat oven to 350 degrees. Line muffin cups with paper liners. If you choose not to use muffin liners, then spray cups with cooking spray.

Mix all dry ingredients together in one bowl. In a separate bowl, mix wet ingredients together. With mixer on low, pour wet ingredients into the dry ones, and stir until they are just blended. Spoon the batter into the cups, filling each one just to the top. Bake for 30 minutes. Ensure doneness by inserting toothpick and removing it; the toothpick should come out clean.

BRIOCHE

YIELDS 16 2¼-OUNCE À TÊTE (WITH HEAD) SERVINGS AT 35 MG PER SERVING

5 fl. ounces whole milk

2¼ ounces granulated sugar

3 large eggs

1 Tbsp. kosher salt

0.6 Tbsp. instant yeast

1 lb. bread flour

13 Tbsp. plus 2 tsp. butter (softened)

1 tsp. clean cannabis butter
(reference recipe)

INSTRUCTIONS

Combine milk and sugar. Add whisked eggs. Combine the yeast in with the flour; add to the wet ingredients. Then add salt. Knead for 5 to 6 minutes. Add softened butter in piece by piece. Knead until butter is incorporated. Ferment overnight in the refrigerator. Scale into the appropriate weight according to the size of the mold. Butter 2 8x4 loaf pans. Divide dough into 2 equal pieces. Divide each piece into 8 equal pieces; form each piece into a ball. Place 8 balls of dough in each loaf pan, side-by-side and proof.*
Egg wash and bake at 375 degrees (internal temperature 200 degrees) until golden brown.

* **Proof:** Proofing dough refers to the final rise of shaped bread before baking. It references a specific rest period within the more generalized process known as fermentation. Allow your brioche dough to proof for 1 ½–2 hours in a warm place without draughts and cover with a clean kitchen towel. This prevents a crust from forming.

KALE PESTO/WHITE SAUCE PIZZA

YIELDS 12 SERVINGS AT 21.5 MG PER SERVING

¾ cup warm water (105 to 115 degrees)

1 packet active yeast

2 cups all-purpose flour

1 tsp. sugar

¾ tsp. salt

2 Tbsp. olive oil

1 Tbsp. cannabis oil

KALE PESTO

2 cups kale (torn without stems)

1 cup fresh packed basil

1 tsp. salt

3 Tbsp. olive oil and 1 tsp. olive oil

1 tsp. cannabis oil (reference recipe)

¼ cup walnuts (blanched)

4 cloves garlic

½ cup parmesan cheese

PARMESAN WHITE SAUCE

2 tsp. butter

1 tsp. clean cannabis butter (reference recipe)

1 medium onion (chopped)

1 clove garlic (finely chopped)

1 Tbsp. flour

½ cup vegetable broth

⅓ cup milk

1 tsp. basil

¼ cup grated parmesan cheese

INSTRUCTIONS

Preheat oven to 350 degrees.

Pour water into small bowl and stir in yeast. Let stand 5 minutes until yeast dissolves. Brush large mixing bowl with olive oil and set aside. Mix flour, sugar, and salt. Add yeast mixture, olive oil, and cannabis oil. Process until dough forms into a sticky ball. Knead dough on lightly floured surface until smooth for about 1 minute (add Tbsp. of flour if your dough is too sticky). Place dough in the prepared bowl, turning dough so that it is coated with oil. Cover bowl with plastic wrap and let it rise in warm area until it is double the size, about 1 hour. Roll out dough, starting in the center of dough and working outwards towards the edge. Do not roll over the edges, because you want to be sure to have a nice crust.

In a food processor, combine the kale leaves, basil leaves, and salt. Pulse until the kale leaves are finely chopped. With the motor running, drizzle in the olive oil. Add the walnuts and garlic and process again, and then add the cheese and pulse to combine.

Cook for 20 minutes.

BUD PAIRING: If you're gonna go with a white sauce, it's only apropos that you go with White Cheese. DANK! This strain has a skunky aroma with earthy tones that will leave you feeling relaxed.

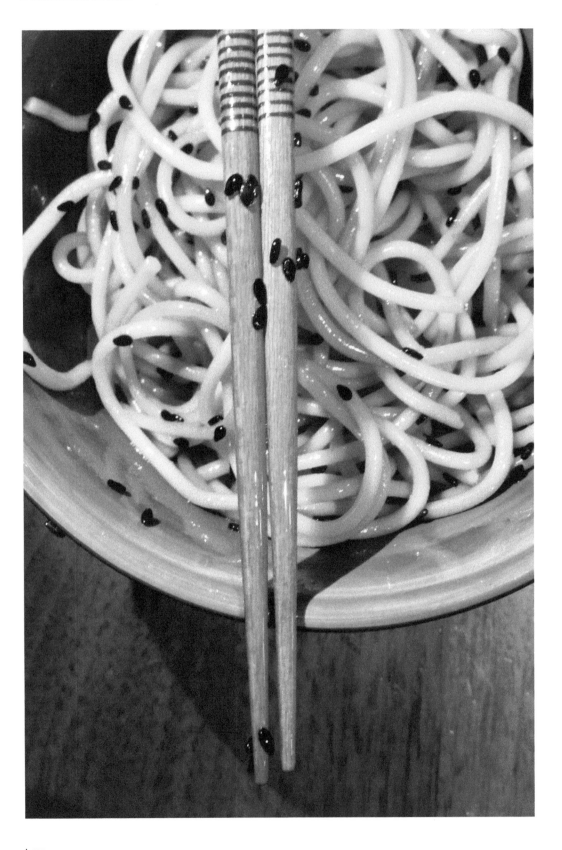

SESAME NOODLES

YIELDS 4 SERVINGS AT 11.7 MG PER SERVING

¾ lb. dried rice noodles

2 Tbsp. toasted sesame oil

1 Tbsp. white miso paste

½ Tbsp. creamy peanut butter

3½ Tbsp. soy sauce

2 Tbsp. rice vinegar

1 Tbsp. brown sugar

1 Tbsp. grated ginger (fine)

3 tsp. minced garlic

Black sesame seeds to garnish

1 tsp. cannabis chili oil (reference recipe)

INSTRUCTIONS

Cook noodles according to package directions, then rinse with cold water to cool. Drain well. Drizzle with a tiny splash of toasted sesame oil to keep them from sticking until dressed.

Meanwhile, whisk miso paste and peanut butter in the bottom of a small bowl, then whisk in soy sauce, rice vinegar, remaining 2 Tbsp. sesame oil, sugar, ginger, garlic, and cannabis chili oil to taste until smooth. Adjust flavors to taste. Toss sauce with cold noodles.

Place in bowl, garnish with sesame seeds.

SAVORY CARIBBEAN HAND PIE

YIELDS 10 SERVINGS AT 30.63 MG PER SERVING

1 lb. callaloo (washed)

1 Tbsp. butter

2 medium chopped onions

Salt to taste

¼ cup water

1 clove garlic

1 Scotch Bonnet hot pepper (for spicy version)

1 Tbsp. black pepper

2 tsp. cannabis oil (reference recipe)

1 cup water

PIE CRUST

2 cups flour

2 tsp. turmeric

½ tsp. salt

3 Tbsp. butter

1 Tbsp. clean cannabis butter (reference recipe)

¼ cup shortening

⅓ cup water

INSTRUCTIONS

Cut up callaloo leaves in pieces. Sauté chopped onion, pepper, & garlic in butter (Add scotch bonnet for spicy version) Add cut up callaloo leaves, water, cannabis oil and stir. Sprinkle with pepper and salt. Cover saucepan and cook callaloo for 7 minutes. Do not overcook. Remove from stovetop and let it cool.

Make the crust: Combine flour, 1½ tsp. curry powder, and pinch of salt. Cut in ¼ cup butter and shortening until mixture resembles coarse crumbs. Stir in water until mixture forms a ball. Do not over stir; that makes tough crust. Shape dough into a log, and cut into 10 equal sections. Roll each section into a 6-inch circle (approximately ⅛-inch thick). Set aside.

Assembling Caribbean Hand Pie: Scoop a heaping Tbsp. of filling into each circle, and brush with egg white around half of the circle. Fold over and seal by pressing the tines of a fork along the edges of the dough.

Preheat oven to 375 degrees.

Place each pie on a baking sheet and bake for about 30 minutes. Serve warm.

BUD PAIRING: Pasties are to islanders what tacos are to Mexicans. In paying homage to my Jamaican roots, I like to use Lambs Breath with this dish. This strain is known as an heirloom because it has distinct roots in a certain region. Lamb's Breath will have you happy, uplifted, and energetic; much like the island of Jamaica.

BARNYARD AND FARM ANIMALS

The interesting thing about tradition is how it shapes one's perceptions and ideas about the world, from politics, to celebrities, to how we adorn ourselves and our food. Traditions validate our culture and inform others about who we are. As vital as it is to preserve cultural traditions, they can also serve a purpose in the blending, bending, and elevating of cultures.

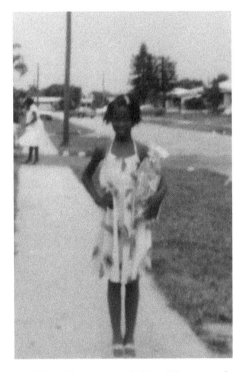

Tradition is as important to my family as apple pie is to American culture. Take Easter, for example– every spring brought April, and every April brought Easter Sunday. With Easter Sunday came a number of absolutes: you would absolutely be in church all day, and an egg hunt would absolutely be pending. You would hunt for water-colored eggs wearing the absolute finest of frilly dresses, opaque stockings, and uncomfortable patent leather shoes.

Somewhere around the age of 10, I decided to break rank. My mother and I scoured the racks of several department stores, all presenting their finest in pink layered taffeta, ruffles, bows, and bonnets. I wanted nothing from this collection of "look at me, I look like you" holiday apparel. But I humored mother. She held up different dresses, reminding me that all of the young ladies at church would be twirling in similar ones. I resisted heaving and found something wrong with all of them. "I don't like the sleeves on that one." "The hem is wrong on this one." "That color! I just can't wear it!" Suffice to say, we were both exhausted.

We went off in different directions to cool ourselves down. A few racks later, my sight landed on the perfect holiday dress for me, a single layered sundress that tied around the neck. It was white with, I kid you not, mouthwatering watermelon slices dotting its entire length. I was thrilled. I snatched up the dress, smiling broadly, and marched over to my mother. I held it high and proudly proclaimed, "This one!"

Though she finally acquiesced, 35 years later, she still gives me shit about it! I had spat in the face of tradition. I had shown up to Sunday service sans lace, gloves, pomp, or circumstance. Her child was the one wearing the watermelon-ridden sundress!

I came to understand that the very idea of my moving away from tradition was scary for my mother. Breaking from the familiar was synonymous with death or extinction. There was no compromise.

What I would hope for her now is to know that the thought of *not exploring other ideals beyond the familiar was and is* just as terrifying for me. I believe that in the place of curiosity, exploration, bending, blending, and elevating, we become one with humanity. We can trust that the foundation is solid, and we can strike a balance between tradition and inclusion.

In these recipes, you'll see my curiosity manifest. May it be as exciting for you as life is to me.

CHICKEN MARSALA

YIELDS 4 SERVINGS AT 12.5 MG PER SERVING

4 boneless skinless chicken thighs

All-purpose flour

Extra virgin olive oil (as needed)

Kosher salt to taste

Black pepper to taste

¼ tsp. aged balsamic vinegar

8 ounces baby belle mushrooms (sliced)

2 cloves garlic (minced)

1 shallot (minced)

¾ cup Marsala wine

¾ cup chicken stock

Fresh parsley to garnish

½ tsp. cornstarch

1 tsp. clean cannabis butter
(reference recipe)

Chopped parsley

INSTRUCTIONS

Add 2½ Tbsp. of olive oil to skillet heated to medium-high. In a bowl, mix flour and salt and pepper to taste. Dredge chicken in flour, shaking off excess.

Once the skillet is hot, add chicken and sear on both sides, about 5–7 minutes per side. Chicken should be golden and cooked through. Add oil if needed. Transfer chicken to a clean plate.

Lower temperature to the skillet and add mushrooms. Cook for about 2 minutes until mushrooms slightly caramelize. Add garlic and finely minced shallots. Cook until the shallots are translucent. Deglaze the pan with the masala wine, and increase the heat slightly. Reduce to about one third original volume of liquid. Add balsamic and cook for another 2–5 minutes.

Add chicken stock and lower the heat. Allow the combination to simmer for about 10 minutes. Add clean cannabis butter. Stir until butter is fully incorporated into the sauce. The sauce will naturally thicken. However, for a richer, thicker consistency, you can opt to whisk together one-third cup of water with the cornstarch (optional). Season to taste with kosher salt and black pepper. Place the chicken back into the skillet.

Simmer until chicken is warmed through. Garnish with chopped parsley.

Traditionally, Chicken Marsala is served over pasta al dente. A version of this dish is presented in southern cuisine and is called Smothered Chicken. As in the Chicken Marsala, mushrooms can be replaced with caramelized onions; however, it is traditionally served with rice or mashed potatoes.

 BUD PAIRING: The depth of this rich sauce pairs favorably with the popular strain Northern Lights. This earthy and sweet indica compliments the Marsala wine and sautéed mushrooms or caramelized onions. Whichever direction you choose, you can't go wrong with this cannabis strain.

PORK CROQUETTES WITH PLANTAIN SALSA AND CHIPOTLE AIOLI

YIELDS 8 SERVINGS AT 6.7 MG PER CROQUETTE

PORK CROQUETTES:

2½ lbs. pork shoulder

3 large oranges

2 large blood oranges

4 limes

1 head of garlic

Cumin

1 Scotch Bonnet/Habanero pepper

1 cup of orange juice

Olive oil as needed

Dried oregano

Chicken stock

Peppercorns

2 bay leaves

1 bunch cilantro (washed)

3 eggs

4 cups panko breadcrumbs

2 cups flour

Canola oil

1 Tbsp. garlic roasted cannabis oil (reference recipe)

1 tsp. cannabis oil (reference recipe)

Kosher salt

1 tsp. paprika

½ tsp. onion powder

1½ Tbsp. brown sugar

PLANTAIN SALSA:

3 ripe plantains (diced)

3 Tbsp. red onion (diced)

2 Roma tomatoes (peeled, seeded and diced)

2 garlic cloves (minced fine)

1 ½ Tbsp. chopped cilantro

Salt and Pepper to taste

Olive Oil

¼ tsp. Habanero or Scotch Bonnet peppers (finely diced – optional)

INSTRUCTIONS

Preheat oven to 350 degrees.

Peel oranges, blood oranges, and limes and then cut in half. Set peels aside. In a medium-sized, oven friendly stockpot, bring 3 Tbsp. of olive oil to a medium-high heat. Brown the pork shoulder on all sides. Remove pork shoulder and set aside, then add orange and lime peels. Cook until fragrant. Add head of garlic, peppercorns, bay leaves, cumin, Scotch Bonnet or Habanero peppers, onion powder, paprika, dried oregano, and a bunch of cilantro. Cook until the cilantro is wilted and the pot is extremely fragrant. Lower the temperature and squeeze the juice of the oranges, blood oranges, and limes. Simmer for 3 minutes, and then add citrus juices. Place the pork back in the pot and add chicken stock until the pork is completely covered. Cover the pot and place in oven, and cook for about 1½–2 hours. The meat should be fork tender.

Remove the head of garlic from the pot and set aside. Remove the pork as well and set side, allowing it to cool. Strain the liquid, placing it in a small stockpot. Bring to a high heat and add brown sugar. Allow the liquid to boil for about 1 minute, and then bring it down to a low heat. Reduce to about half starting volume.

Once the pork is cool, gently pull and do a rough chop. Take 4 cloves of garlic from the head that was set aside, and mash thoroughly. Add 2–3 Tbsp. of the reduced liquid, the garlic roasted cannabis oil, the infused oil, and 1 beaten egg. Mix thoroughly. Incorporate the wet ingredients into the pulled pork. Add salt and pepper if needed.

Portion and shape the mixture in 4-ounce patties. Place in the refrigerator, and allow them to set for a minimum of 3 hours.

In a medium-sized stockpot, bring the canola oil to a steady temperature of 350 degrees. Meanwhile, prepare a dredge of seasoned flour in a bowl. In a separate bowl, whisk the remaining eggs with 3 Tbsp. of water. Place the panko breadcrumbs in a third bowl.

Dredge the patties first in seasoned flour, then in the egg, and finally the breadcrumbs. Deep-fry the croquettes until they are golden brown. Serve with plantain salsa and chipotle aioli.

PLANTAIN SALSA

In a medium-sized skillet, bring to a medium-high heat, about 3 Tbsp. of olive oil. Fry ripened diced plantains until they are golden. Allow them to drain and cool slightly. Mix with chopped cilantro, diced tomato, onion powder, minced garlic, red onion, salt/pepper to taste, diced Habanero/Scotch Bonnet pepper, and 1 Tbsp. of olive oil. Mix gently and serve with pork croquettes.

For an enhanced version of the salsa, substitute this for the olive oil.

CHIPOTLE AIOLI

*6 Tbsp. infused mayonnaise
(reference infused mayonnaise recipe)*

2 Tbsp. chipotle in adobo (chopped fine)

1 tsp. garlic (minced)

½ tsp. cumin

4 tsp. lemon juice

Kosher salt to taste

INSTRUCTIONS

Blend all ingredients in small food processor. Transfer to a bowl or squeeze bottle and refrigerate.

INFUSED MAYONNAISE

YIELDS 12 SERVINGS AT 11.7 MG PER SERVING

1 large egg yolk

1½ tsp. fresh lemon juice

1 tsp. white wine vinegar

¼ tsp. Dijon mustard

½ tsp. salt plus more to taste

11 Tbsp. California olive oil, divided

1 Tbsp. infused cannabis oil (reference recipe)

INSTRUCTIONS

Combine egg yolk, lemon juice, vinegar, mustard, and ½ tsp. salt in medium bowl. Whisk until blended and bright yellow, about 30 seconds. Using ¼ tsp. measure and whisking constantly, add ¼ cup oil (combine 1 Tbsp. cannabis oil and 3 Tbsp. olive oil) to yolk mixture a few drops at a time, over about 4 minutes. Gradually add remaining ½ cup olive oil in very slow thin stream, whisking constantly, until mayonnaise is thick, about 8 minutes (mayonnaise will be lighter in color). Cover and chill.

SALISBURY STEAK WITH TWICE COOKED POTATOES & ONION GRAVY

YIELDS 6 PATTIES AT 23 MG PER SERVING

1 lb. ground beef

½ lb. braised beef (pulled)

¼ cup nutritional yeast flakes

1 egg (beaten)

2 cloves garlic (minced)

½ tsp. fresh thyme

1 Tbsp. steak seasoning

¼ tsp. horseradish

Bacon fat

Kosher salt and freshly ground black pepper to taste

BROWN ONION GRAVY:

2–3 large red onions (thinly sliced)

3 cups beef stock

½ cup dry red wine

1 Tbsp. tomato paste

2 Tbsp. corn starch

1 Tbsp. clarified butter (reference recipe)

2 tsp. clean cannabis butter (reference recipe)

Kosher salt and freshly ground black pepper to taste

INSTRUCTIONS

Combine the ground beef, braised beef, nutritional yeast flakes, egg, garlic, horseradish, steak seasoning, thyme, and salt and pepper to taste. Shape the meat mixture into 6 equal sized patties.

Heat clean cannabis butter and olive oil in large sauté pan. Add onions and cook over medium-high heat for approximately 20 minutes until onions start to caramelize, stirring occasionally.

Add ¼ cup of the beef stock and continue cooking, stirring for another 10 minutes. Add wine and reduce liquid by half. Stir in the remaining beef stock, tomato paste, and salt and pepper to taste.

Simmer for another 10 minutes. Combine ⅛ of a cup of cold water with all-purpose flour or cornstarch. Add as needed until the gravy reaches the desired consistency. Reduce heat to the lowest temperature to keep warmed through.

Heat the bacon fat in a large skillet over a medium-high heat. Sear patties 2–4 minutes per side. For added flavor, grill the patties for an additional minute per side or until each form grill marks. Return the patties to the skillet, and pour the gravy over the patties and simmer for an additional 10 minutes.

QUAIL CONFIT WITH BALSAMIC BLUEBERRY BBQ SAUCE

YIELDS 6 SERVINGS AT 14.1 MG PER SERVING

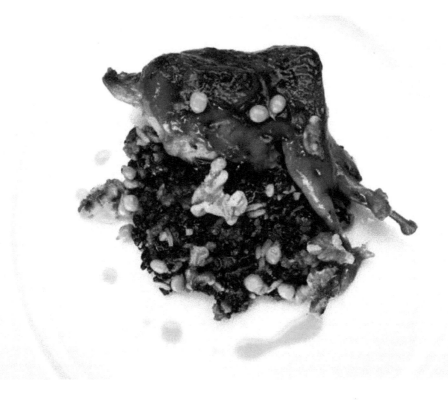

6 quails

12 cloves of garlic

6 sprigs of thyme

3 tsp. of garlic powder

3 tsp. kosher salt

1 quart of duck fat

INSTRUCTIONS

Preheat oven to 340 degrees. Season each quail with equal parts garlic powder and kosher salt. Stuff each quail with 2 cloves of garlic and 1 sprig of thyme. Truss each quail so that the thyme and garlic remain inside of the bird. Place quails in a 2–3-inch baking pan and fully submerge with the duck fat. Cook for 1 hour or until fork-tender. Remove from the oven and allow to cool.

Gently remove quail from duck fat and transfer to draining station. Pat dry and refrigerate while preparing barbecue sauce.

Once barbecue sauce is complete, place quail on baking sheet and brush generously with sauce. Place in preheated oven of 300 degrees. As barbecue sauce begins to caramelize, continue coating with additional sauce. Repeat for up to 30 minutes until the sauce is evenly distributed.

BLUEBERRY BBQ SAUCE

YIELDS 8 SERVINGS AT 2 OUNCES AND 18.75 MG PER SERVING

2 cups fresh blueberries

1 8-ounce can tomato sauce

½ cup balsamic vinegar

⅓ cup honey

¼ cup tomato paste

¼ cup molasses

3 Tbsp. Worcestershire sauce

2 tsp. liquid smoke

1 tsp. smoked paprika

2 cloves minced garlic

½ tsp. black pepper

½ tsp. onion powder

½ tsp. salt

1 Tbsp. cannabis oil (reference recipe)

INSTRUCTIONS

Whisk all ingredients together in medium saucepan. Bring to simmer over medium-high heat. Reduce heat to medium low and simmer (uncovered) for 20 minutes, or until the sauce has thickened. Place in blender and blend until smooth.

BUD PAIRING: To fortify the flavor of the barbecue sauce, I went with the obvious pairing of Blueberry Kush. This indica-dominant hybrid elevates the natural sweetness of the blueberry barbecue sauce. As well, its medicinal effects will lead to a restful night after this comfort meal.

STUFFED PORK CHOP WITH WHITE WINE DIJON SAUCE

YIELDS 6 SERVINGS AT 14.1 MG PER SERVING

¼ cup kosher salt

3 Tbsp. raw sugar

2 quarts water

4 sprigs of rosemary

2 oranges

1 head of garlic (cut in half lengthwise)

6 2-inch boneless pork chops

1 Tbsp. extra virgin olive oil

1 Tbsp. butter

½ cup thick cut smoked ham (diced)

½ cup diced onion

1 Tbsp. garlic (minced)

1 tsp. fresh rosemary (chopped fine)

½ tsp. fresh sage (chopped fine)

½ tsp. fresh thyme (chopped fine)

2 Tbsp. freshly chopped parsley leaves

½ Tbsp. clean cannabis butter (reference recipe)

½ Tbsp. garlic roasted cannabis oil (reference recipe)

2½ cups house made croutons

⅔ cup diced apples

⅓ cup toasted walnuts

½ cup chicken broth for dressing

½ cup chicken broth for making pan gravy

Kosher salt and black pepper

DIJON WINE SAUCE :

1 Tbsp. butter

1 Tbsp. olive oil

Salt to taste

Pepper to taste

1 onion (sliced)

2 Tbsp. Dijon mustard

1 cup white wine (Pinot Grigio)

Juice of ½ lemon

1 sprig thyme

1 clove garlic (grated or finely minced)

INSTRUCTIONS

Add pork chops to a brine of 2 quarts of cold water, 3 Tbsp. of brown sugar, 2 oranges, 4 sprigs of rosemary, head of garlic, and a quarter cup of kosher salt. Place in the refrigerator for a minimum of 2 hours.

In a medium skillet, bring about 1 Tbsp. of olive oil to a medium-high heat. Add ham and cook until caramelized. Add in onions, and cook until they are soft. Then add garlic, clean cannabis butter, and garlic roasted cannabis oil. Cook until the onions become translucent. Lightly season with kosher salt and black pepper to taste. Add chopped herb, sauté, and remove from the heat to cool.

Remove the pork chops from the brine and pat dry. Make an incision in each chop, creating a perfect pocket for the stuffing.

In a large bowl, add homemade croutons, diced apples, toasted walnuts, ham/onion mixture, and a half cup of chicken broth. Mix well. Add additional broth by the tsp. and only if necessary. The mixture should not be too soft. Stuff each chop with half a cup of stuffing. Using kitchen grade twine, truss each chop to secure the stuffing. Season each with kosher salt.

On medium-high heat, preheat about a Tbsp. of olive oil in the pan. When hot, place chops in pan and cook until the internal temperature reaches 145 degrees (about 7 minutes per side). For perfection, you can sear the sides to a golden crispness. Use tongs to lift the chops, remove the chops to a plate, and allow them to rest for 5 minutes before serving. This will allow the juices to redistribute rather than running out all over your plate and giving you dry meat.

DIJON SAUCE INSTRUCTIONS

Using the same pan that you cooked the chops in, heat butter and olive oil over medium-high heat. Lower heat to medium-low and add onions. With pan over medium-low heat, carefully pour in cup of white wine and deglaze the bottom of the pan. Add Dijon mustard, thyme leaves, lemon juice, and garlic, and stir to create a sauce.

RAVIOLI WITH BRAISED LAMB AND LOCAL MUSHROOMS

YIELDS 6 SERVINGS AT 22.2 MG PER SERVING

FILLING INGREDIENTS:

1 tsp. garlic roasted cannabis oil (reference recipe)

1 clove garlic (minced)

½ cup onion (chopped)

⅓ cup grated parmesan cheese

1 cup ricotta cheese

1 Tbsp. fresh parsley (chopped)

½ tsp. thyme (chopped)

Salt and ground black pepper to taste

1 egg white (beaten)

3 Tbsp. butter

1 Tbsp. lemon zest

BRAISED LAMB INGREDIENTS

1½ lbs. lamb shank

2 lbs. of assorted mushrooms (oyster, shitake, morel, etc.)

1 onion (roughly chopped)

1 sprig thyme

1 sprig rosemary

1 Tbsp. tomato paste

1 tsp. ground fennel

1 Tbsp. roasted beef base

1 cup of red wine

1 head of garlic

2 bay leaves

1 Tbsp. of white peppercorns

32 ounces veal stock

16 ounces infused mushroom stock (reference recipe)

1 tsp. clean cannabis butter (reference recipe)

2 Tbsp. cream

Canola oil as needed

1 ½ cups all-purpose flour

FILLING INSTRUCTIONS

Heat 1 tsp. olive oil in a skillet over medium heat. Stir in the garlic and onion; cook and stir until the onion begins to soften, about 2 minutes. Remove from heat, and allow to cool.

Mix the cooled onion with the garlic, ricotta cheese, parmesan cheese, spinach, and parsley. Season with salt and pepper.

Roll the pasta dough (see referenced instructions) out to about 1/16 inch thick. Cut 3" to 4-inch circles using a large cookie cutter. Roll each circle out as thin as possible. Working with 1 circle at a time, brush the pasta lightly with the egg white. Scoop about 1 heaping Tbsp. full of the filling onto the center of the pasta, then cover with a second piece of pasta, pinching the edges to seal. Cut the sealed ravioli with the cookie cutter once more to create a uniform shape. Place the finished ravioli on a floured baking sheet, and repeat the process with the remaining pasta and filling.

Fill a large pot with lightly salted water and bring to a rolling boil over high heat. Once the water is boiling, stir in the ravioli and return to a boil. Cook until the pasta floats to the top, 3 to 4 minutes; drain.

INSTRUCTIONS FOR BRAISE:

Place oil in large pot and heat on medium-high. Dredge lamb shanks in flour and shake off the excess. Sear on all sides until browned. Remove. Cook onions and seasonings until onions become translucent. Add tomato paste and stir. Deglaze pan with wine, and then add all liquids. Insert meat, tightly cover the pot, and braise 3 hours on medium low heat. Remove lamb shanks and set aside. Strain the liquid into a saucepan, and reduce until it coats the back of a spoon. Season to taste, add mushrooms until slightly limp, and add cannabis butter and cream. Stir until smooth. Remove from heat and adjust seasoning as need. Add lamb shank (bone removed) to sauce.

BUD PAIRING: I wanted a flavor profile that would stand up to the gaminess of the lamb yet complement the earthy notes of the mushrooms and still allow the subtlety of the cheese-filled pasta to shine through. For this reason, I paired Cali Kush, a local favorite known for its fruity citrus aroma and coffee notest.

CHICKEN POT PIE

YIELDS 6 SERVINGS AT 14.1 MG PER SERVING

4 cups chicken broth

1 bouillon cube

½ cup (1 stick) butter

1 tsp. clean cannabis butter (reference recipe)

1 onion (finely chopped)

2 large carrots (diced)

2 cloves garlic (chopped fine)

Salt and freshly ground black pepper

½ cup all-purpose flour

¼ cup heavy cream

3 Tbsp. white wine

2 lbs. roasted chicken, shredded (reference recipe below)

18 ounces broccoli florets

Pie dough (reference recipe)

1 egg beaten with 1 Tbsp. water

ROASTED CHICKEN INGREDIENTS:

2 lb. whole chicken

½ Tbsp. minced garlic

1 tsp. clean cannabis butter (reference recipe)

½ stick butter (room temperature)

1 Tbsp. tarragon (chopped fine)

1 Tbsp. thyme (chopped fine)

Kosher salt to taste

4 cloves garlic

1 sprig rosemary

2 sprigs thyme

1 bay leaf

PIE CRUST INGREDIENTS:

2½ cups all-purpose flour

1 tsp. salt

2 Tbsp. sugar

¾ cup (a stick and a half) unsalted butter, chilled, cut into 1/4 inch cubes

½ cup of all-vegetable shortening (8 Tbsp.)

6–8 Tbsp. ice water

INSTRUCTIONS FOR PIE CRUST:

Combine flour, salt, and sugar in a food processor; pulse to mix. Add the butter and pulse 4 times. Add shortening in Tbsp. sized chunks, and pulse 4 more times. The mixture should resemble coarse cornmeal, with butter bits no bigger than peas. Sprinkle 6 Tbsp. of ice water over flour mixture. Pulse a couple times. If you pinch some of the crumbly dough and it holds together, it's ready. If the dough doesn't hold together, keep adding water, a Tbsp. at a time, pulsing once after each addition, until the mixture just begins to clump together.

Remove dough from machine and place in a mound on a clean surface. Divide the dough into 2 balls and flatten each into

4-inch wide disks. Do not over-knead the dough! Dust the disks lightly with flour, wrap each in plastic, and refrigerate for at least an hour, or for up to 2 days, before rolling out.

After the dough has chilled in the refrigerator for an hour, you can take it out to roll. If it is too stiff, you may need to let it sit for 5–10 minutes at room temperature before rolling. Sprinkle a little flour on a flat, clean work surface and on top of the disk of dough you intend to roll out.

INSTRUCTIONS FOR ROASTED CHICKEN:

Preheat oven to 350 degrees. Mix minced garlic, chopped herbs, cannabis butter, and butter. Place the butter mixture carefully between the skin and chicken, being careful not to rip the skin. Stuff the cavity of the bird with sprigs of thyme, rosemary, cloves of garlic, and bay leaf. Season with kosher salt. Truss the legs of the chicken and roast chicken for 1 hour 20 minutes, basting periodically.

INSTRUCTIONS FOR POT PIE:

Preheat your oven to 375 degrees F.

In a large saucepan, heat chicken broth and bouillon over medium heat until hot.

In a separate skillet, melt butter over medium heat; add onions, carrots, and garlic, and sauté until tender. Season with salt and pepper. Add the flour and whisk until there are no lumps. Stir in the hot broth, cream, wine, chicken and broccoli. Bring to a boil, then reduce to a simmer.

With a ladle, fill 6 ovenproof ramekins or bowls with the filling. Place on baking sheet.

Sprinkle flour on countertop. Roll out dough an extra inch. Using a biscuit round or mold, cut out dough to cover the tops of your ramekins, with about half an inch hanging over, depending on their size. Crimp the dough over the edge of the ramekin. Brush with the egg wash and make small slits on the top. Bake for 35 minutes. Remove from the oven and serve.

JERK CHICKEN

YIELDS 4 SERVINGS AT 23.5 MG PER SERVING

4 chicken breasts

½ cup malt vinegar

2 Tbsp. dark rum

*2 Scotch Bonnet peppers
(or Habaneros), with seeds, chopped*

1 red onion (chopped)

4 green onions (chopped)

2 Tbsp. fresh thyme leaves (chopped)

2 Tbsp. olive oil

2 Tsp. cannabis oil

2 tsp. salt

2 tsp. freshly ground black pepper

4 tsp. ground allspice

4 tsp. ground cinnamon

4 tsp. ground nutmeg

4 tsp. ground ginger

2 tsp. molasses

½ cup lime juice

Salt and pepper

INSTRUCTIONS

Put vinegar, rum, hot peppers, onion, green onion tops, thyme, olive oil, salt, pepper, allspice, cinnamon, nutmeg, ginger, and molasses into a blender. Pulse until mostly smooth.

Place chicken in a large bowl and pour lime juice over the chicken, making sure to coat well. Season with jerk sauce, cover bowl with plastic, and refrigerate overnight.

When you are ready to cook the chicken, remove it from the marinade bowl and place on grill.

Preheat grill to medium-high. Sprinkle chicken breasts with salt and pepper. Place chicken on grill. Cover. Cook for approximately 30 minutes, keeping the internal grill temperature between 350°F and 400°F, turning the chicken occasionally and basting with marinade, until the chicken is cooked through.

While chicken is grilling: put the remaining marinade into a small saucepan. Bring to a boil, reduce heat and simmer for 10 minutes. Set aside to use as a basting sauce for the chicken. This sauce can even be used as a dressing.

Serve with rice and peas.

STEAK AU POIVRE

YIELDS 4 SERVINGS AT 14.1 MG PER SERVING

4 filet mignon (8-10 ounces each)

1 Tbsp. kosher salt

2 Tbsp. whole red peppercorns

1 Tbsp. vegetable oil

⅓ cup finely chopped shallots

½ stick (1/4 cup) unsalted butter, cut into 4 pieces

2 tsp. cannabis butter (reference recipe)

½ cup Hennessy or other cognac

¾ cup heavy cream

INSTRUCTIONS

Preheat oven to 200°F.

Pat steaks dry and season both sides with kosher salt.

Coarsely crush peppercorns, and coat pepper evenly onto both sides of steaks.

Heat a 12-inch heavy skillet (preferably cast-iron) over moderately high heat until hot, about 3 minutes, then add oil, swirling skillet, and sauté steaks in 2 batches, turning over once, about 6 minutes per batch for medium rare steaks.

Transfer steaks as cooked to a heatproof platter and keep warm in oven while making sauce.

Pour off fat from skillet, and then add shallots and add cannabis butter and half of butter (2 Tbsp.) to skillet; cook over moderately low heat, stirring and scraping up brown bits, until shallots are well-browned all over, 3-5 minutes.

Add Hennessy (use caution; it may ignite) and boil, stirring, until liquid is reduced to a glaze, 2 to 3 minutes. Add cream and any meat juices accumulated on platter, and boil sauce, stirring occasionally, until reduced by half, 3 to 5 minutes. Add remaining 2 Tbsp. butter and cook over low heat, swirling skillet, until butter is incorporated. Serve sauce with steaks.

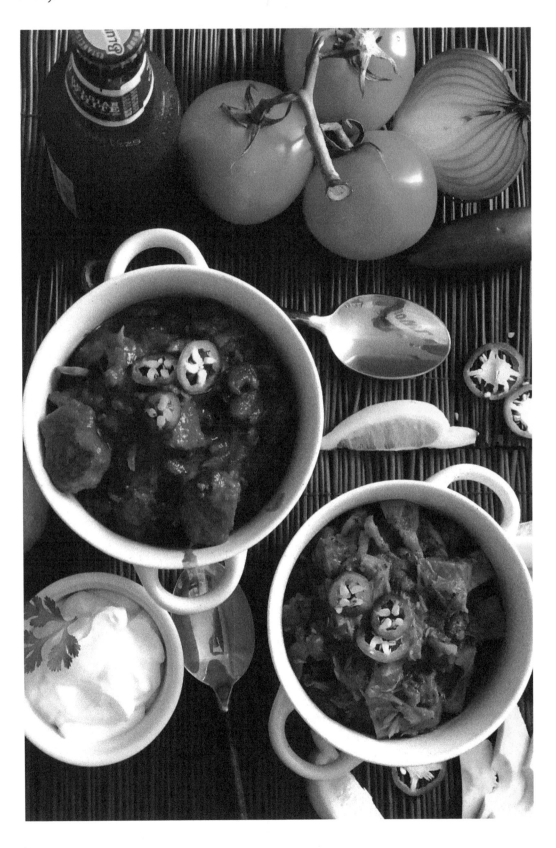

BEEF & BISON SPICY CHILI

YIELDS 6 SERVINGS AT 16.6 MG PER SERVING

½ lb. bison (cubed)

½ lb. ground sirloin

¼ lb. pork shoulder (cubed)

2 onions (diced)

1 green peppers, diced

1 Tbsp. jalapeño, finely chopped

14 ounces heirloom tomatoes (diced)

8 ounces tomato sauce

6 ounces tomato paste

2 Tbsp. cumin

1 Tbsp. fresh oregano (chopped fine)

¼ Tbsp. rosemary (chopped fine)

2 Tbsp. powder

1 tsp. salt

½ tsp. cayenne pepper

½ tsp. smoked paprika

½ tsp. garlic powder

1 bay leaf

14 ounce can kidney beans

14 ounce can black beans

1 cup water

1 cup veal or beef stock (more as needed)

1 gram cannabis sachet

INSTRUCTIONS

In large pot heat 3 Tbsp. of olive oil over medium heat. Cook bison, ground sirloin, and pork shoulder with onions and peppers in large pot. Drain excess grease, and add tomatoes, seasonings, water, and veal or beef stock, then bring to a boil. Add beans and sachet, cover, and simmer 1–2 hours. Garnish with sour cream, sliced avocado, and cilantro.

VEGAN SPICY CHILI

YIELDS 6 SERVINGS AT 16.6 MG PER SERVING

1 lb can jackfruit

¼ lb vegan chorizo

2 onions (diced)

1 green peppers (diced)

1 tbsp jalapeno (finely chopped)

14 ounces heirloom tomatoes (diced)

8 ounces tomato sauce

6 ounces tomato paste

2 tbsp cumin

1 Tbsp fresh oregano (chopped fine)

¼ Tbsp rosemary (chopped fine)

2 tbsp chili powder

1 tsp salt

1⁄2 tsp cayenne pepper

1⁄2 tsp smoked paprika

½ tsp garlic powder

1 bay leaf

14 ounce can kidney beans

14 ounce can black beans

1 cup water

1 cup vegetable stock (more as needed)

1 gram cannabis sachet

Vegan sour cream

INSTRUCTIONS

In a large pot sauté vegan chorizo on medium heat for 7-10 minutes. Add drained jackfruit, onions and peppers. Cook until onions are translucent, then remove from the pot and set aside. Add tomatoes, seasonings, water, and vegetable stock, and then bring to a boil. Add beans and sachet, cover, and simmer 30 minutes and then add the chorizo and jackfruit back to the pot. Simmer for another 15-20 minutes. Garnish with vegan sour cream, sliced avocado, and cilantro.

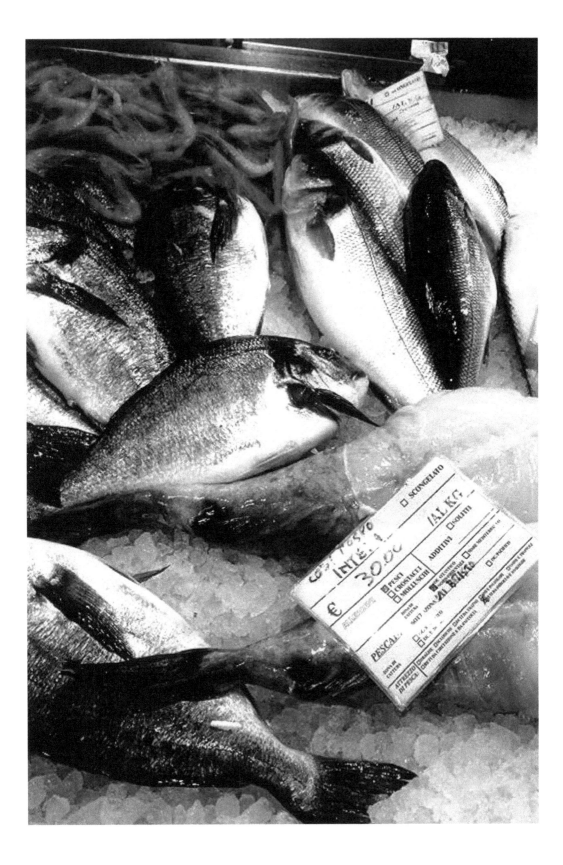

SEAFOOD, SNAILS AND SHELLFISH

*"Give a man a fish and you feed him for a day.
Teach a man to fish and you feed him for a lifetime."*
–Chinese Proverb

Out of necessity and intrigue, I learned to cook. For the very same reasons, I learned to fish. I am from the south.

Often, the proclamation of my southern roots is met with resistance or countered with fantastical tales of south Florida and the 2 Live Crew rap group. The fact remains that Florida *is* the southernmost point of the east coast. If you pair that with my family's migration from the Bible Belt city of Statesboro, Georgia, I can assure you that I definitely hail from the Deep South.

The tale of these two cities is juxtaposed perfectly in my coming-of-age story. In Georgia, I learned to properly shuck corn, snap peas, clean collard greens, and skin a frog. While in Ft. Lauderdale, the DIY way of life translated into throwing out a line, catching, gutting, and scaling a fish. There was crabbing, deep sea fishing, and messing around with eels in shallow streams. I've even pried thirsty leeches from the flesh of my shins after wading through canals. The Florida peninsula provided me with the fruits of the sea and beyond.

In culinary school, my classmates cringed at the idea of cleaning a fish, whereas I was simply bewildered by the tool I was given to do so. As a young-'un, I learned to use a fork while shielding my face with nothing more than a periodic swipe of my shoulder sleeve. So, cooking fish in culinary school was both second nature and foreign to me: the smell of the ocean wafting up from the deep silver prep sink, flying scales, discarded innards, and then this new tool. In one moment, I realized that what I most appreciate about cooking seafood is the direct interaction involved in its preparation. We don't usually have to stare down an entire cow, pig, or chicken before making it our dinner. We buy it faceless, quartered, sliced, chopped, ground or deboned. But with seafood—think wild-caught prawns or farm-raised catfish—we often buy it complete with eyes, whiskers, and tails.

My belief is that if you cannot look it in the face and honor its sacrifice, you shouldn't eat it. With that, let's stare down and dig in.

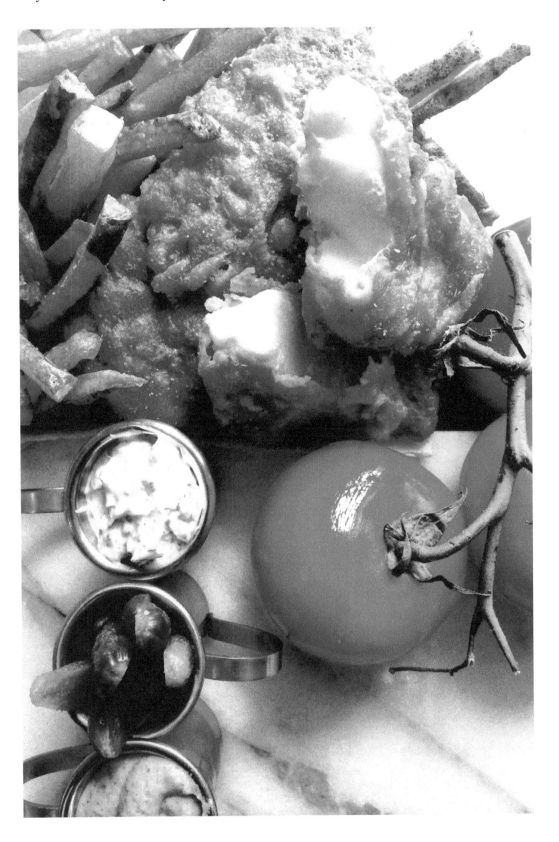

FRIED COD WITH TARTAR SAUCE

YIELDS 4 SERVINGS AT 19.7 MG PER SERVING

INGREDIENTS:

YIELDS 11.7 MG PER SERVING

*½ cup infused mayonnaise
(reference recipe)*

2 Tbsp. cornichons (diced fine)

1 Tbsp. lemon juice

1 Tbsp. thyme (chopped fine)

½ Tbsp. tarragon (chopped fine)

½ tsp. garlic powder

1 tsp. Dijon mustard

Kosher salt (to taste)

8 pieces cod

1½ cup of cornmeal (fine ground)

½ cup all-purpose flour

*1½ Tbsp. of house made lemon pepper
seasoning (reference recipe)*

⅓ cup canola oil

LEMON PEPPER SEASONING

**YIELDS 6 SERVINGS AT 8 MG
PER SERVING**

4 Tbsp. lemon zest

1 Tbsp. ground black peppercorns

1 Tbsp. white peppercorns

½ Tbsp. salt

½ gram of cannabis

INSTRUCTIONS

SEASONING

Mix all ingredients. Place on parchment paper on sheet tray, then bake in the oven at 250 degrees for 20 minutes.

TARTAR SAUCE

Place all the ingredients in a food processor or mini chopper fitted with a steel blade, and pulse several times until the pickles are finely chopped and all the ingredients are well mixed but not pureed.

FISH

Mix dry ingredients (cornmeal, seasoning, and flour). In skillet, bring the canola oil to a high temperature (315 degrees). Rinse fish, dredge in flour/cornmeal mix, and fry fish on both sides until golden brown and cooked through, 1–3 minutes per side depending on thickness of fish. Serve with tartar sauce.

BLACKENED SWORD FISH WITH SMASHED POTATOES

YIELDS 4 SERVINGS AT 17.5 MG PER SERVING

4 pieces of sword fish

4 Tbsp. blackened seasoned infused compound butter (reference recipe)

4 tsp. blackened seasoning

4 tsp. garlic roasted cannabis oil (reference recipe)

1 Tbsp. of cannabis oil (reference recipe)

½ lb. potatoes

1 Tbsp. roasted garlic and chive infused butter (reference recipe)

½ tsp. salt

Cream or milk as needed

INSTRUCTIONS

Season fish. Sear in oil and butter combinations (1/2 Tbsp. per side). Remove, drain, and serve with smashed potatoes.

Potatoes: boil potatoes until soft. Drain, add roasted chive infused butter, cream, and salt and mash up. When you drain potatoes, transfer to bowl and mash immediately–don't allow potatoes to cool.

CAJUN STYLE BAYOU SHRIMP

YIELDS 2 SERVINGS AT 19.79 MG PER SERVING

2 Lbs. shrimp

2 Tbsp. garlic

2 Tbsp. roasted garlic and chive butter (reference recipe)

½ tsp. cannabis oil (reference recipe)

2 Tbsp. olive oil

½ tsp. cayenne pepper

1 tsp. scallions (chopped)

2 Tbsp. parsley

Pinch smoked paprika

1 tsp. house made lemon pepper (reference recipe)

4 Tbsp. white wine

1 tsp. garlic powder

½ tsp. white pepper

1 tsp. fresh thyme (chopped fine)

Kosher salt to taste

INSTRUCTIONS

In a large skillet, heat the cannabis oil and olive oil. Add shrimp and cook until opaque; add all seasonings and mix well. Deglaze with wine. Reduce on lower heat while stirring frequently. Slowly add chilled roasted garlic and chive butter and stir so that sauce emulsifies.

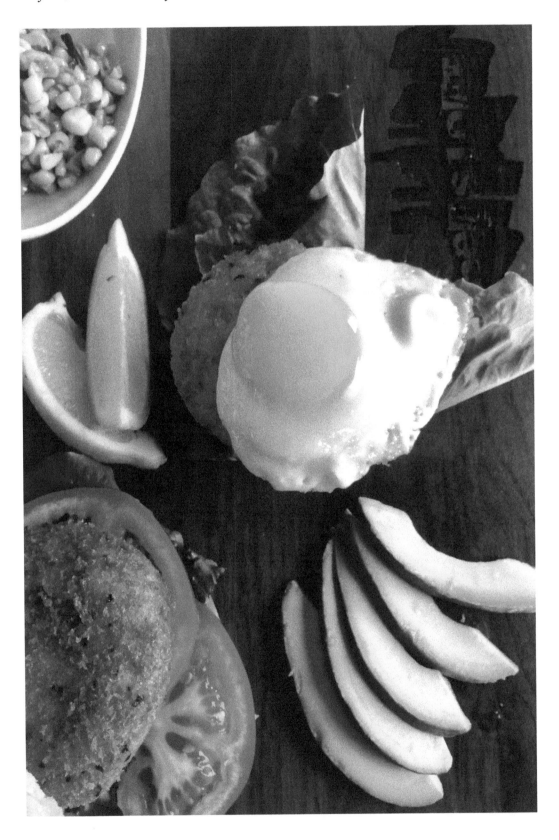

COD CAKE SANDWICHES

YIELDS 4 SERVINGS AT 14.1 MG PER SERVING

1 lb. poached or baked cod fillets
(cooled and flaked)

1 egg

4 potato buns

2 tsp. garlic (minced)

1 Tbsp. thyme

1 tsp. tarragon

½ lemon (juice)

1 ½ Tbsp. of infused mayonnaise
(reference recipe)

½ tsp. cayenne pepper

1 quart oil

DREDGE

2 eggs

2 Tbsp. water

1 ½ cup panko breadcrumbs

1 ½ cups all-purpose flour

½ tsp. kosher salt

INSTRUCTIONS

Take cooked cod and add mayo, thyme, tarragon, lemon juice, and cayenne pepper. Mix and adjust seasoning as needed. Taste. Add 1 beaten egg and mix well. Portion into 4 patties.

Take patties and dredge in all-purpose flour. Dip into egg wash and then dip into panko. Fry in oil until golden brown. Drain. Serve with aioli, avocado, or other garnish of your choice.

GREEN COCONUT CURRY WITH MUSSELS

YIELDS 4 SERVINGS AT 12.5 MG PER SERVING

2 stalks lemon grass

4 Tbsp. vegetable oil

1 Vidalia onions (diced small)

6 cloves garlic (thinly sliced)

6 Tbsp. peeled ginger (chopped fine)

4 Tbsp. cup green curry paste (reference recipe)

2 15-ounce cans coconut milk

4 Tbsp. fish sauce

4 lbs. mussels (scrubbed and debearded)

4 limes, halved

1 cup chopped fresh cilantro

Crusty bread, for serving (optional)

INSTRUCTIONS

Trim the lemongrass, leaving 6 inches at the root end; discard the tops. Smash the stalks and cut into 1-inch pieces.

Heat 4 Tbsp. oil in large stockpot over medium-high heat. Add sliced onions and cook, stirring, until soft, about 5 minutes. Add the garlic, lemongrass, ginger, and curry paste and cook, stirring, until golden, about 2 minutes.

Add coconut milk, fish sauce, and a half cup of water, and bring to a simmer. Add the mussels; cover and cook, stirring occasionally, until the mussels open, about 8 minutes. (Discard any that do not open.) Add the juice of 4 limes and throw the lime halves in. Stir 1 cup cilantro into each. Serve with bread, if desired.

CURRY PASTE

YIELDS 8 SERVINGS AT 12.5 MG PER SERVING

2 tsp. coriander seeds

1 tsp. dry mustard

½ tsp. cumin

8 whole black peppercorns

2 Tbsp. cilantro (rough chopped)

2 tsp. shrimp paste

1½ tsp. kosher salt

1 tsp. ground Kaffir lime leaves

1 tsp. grated lime zest

4 fresh green Thai chilies

6 cloves garlic (rough chopped)

6 small Asian shallots or 2 medium regular shallots (sliced thin)

1½ stalk lemongrass
(trimmed and sliced thin)

6"piece galangal (peeled and sliced thin)

4" ginger (peeled and minced)

1 gram ground cannabis

INSTRUCTIONS

To make the paste: Heat coriander seeds, dry mustard, cumin, and peppercorns in a cast-iron skillet until seeds begin to pop, 1-2 minutes. Let it cool, then place in spice grinder and pulse until finely ground. Set aside until you complete the next steps.

Place cilantro root, shrimp paste, salt, kaffir lime leaves, lime zest, chilies, garlic, shallots, lemongrass, and galangal in a small food processor; pulse until roughly chopped. Add spice mixture.

BUD PAIRING: Hindu Kush is a great pairing for this curry with its subtle sweet and earthy sandalwood aroma. These vivacious aromas are a great accent to the kaffir, chilies, and galangal. Its euphoric yet relaxed properties are perfect for a spicy Thai inspired dinner.

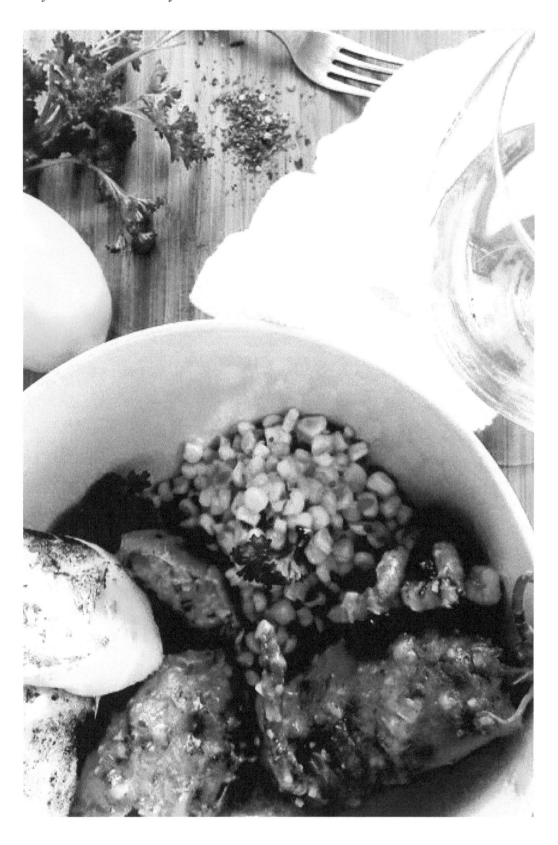

LOBSTER ETOUFFEE

YIELDS 8 SERVINGS AT 14.965 MG PER SERVING

¼ cup oil

¼ cup butter plus 4 Tbsp. butter reserved

½ Tbsp. clean cannabis butter (reference recipe)

½ cup flour, plus extra flour as needed to form a paste

1½ cup yellow onion (chopped)

½ cup green bell pepper (chopped)

3 garlic cloves (minced)

2 bay leaves

½ tsp. white pepper

½ tsp. cayenne pepper or to taste

1 tsp. Cajun seasoning or to taste

3-5 dashes hot sauce or to taste

4 cups lobster stock (reference recipe)

1 14½-ounce can diced tomatoes

1 tsp. salt

4 lobster tails (halved)

½ cup minced green onions, plus extra for garnish

½ cup fresh parsley leaves (minced)

INSTRUCTIONS

To make the roux, melt butter (include cannabis butter at this point) with oil in a large heavy saucepan over low heat. Whisk flour into the oil to form a paste; cook over low heat, whisking continuously until the mixture turns a caramel color and gives off a nutty aroma, about 15 to 20 minutes.

Add the onion, green pepper, and garlic, and cook over low heat until the vegetables are limp, about 5 minutes.

Add the black pepper, white pepper, cayenne pepper, Cajun seasoning, green onions, parsley, and hot sauce to taste. Add lobster stock, tomatoes with their juice, and salt to taste. Bring to a boil, reduce the heat to low, and simmer for 10 to 15 minutes until mixture thickens.

Add lobster and cook for 3–5 minutes, being careful not to overcook. Remove from heat, add the 4 Tbsp. reserved butter, and stir to melt. Garnish with the green onions and parsley and serve over steamed rice.

LOBSTER STOCK

YIELDS 2 QUARTS (64 CUPS) SERVINGS AT 3.43 MG PER 1 CUP

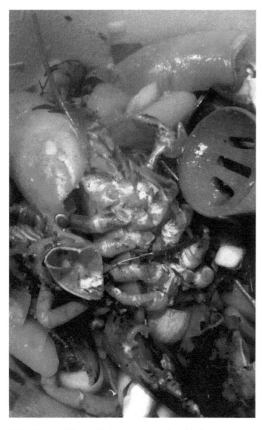

Shells and heads from 4 cooked lobsters

2 large peeled carrots (rough chopped)

2 large onions (rough chopped)

4 Tbsp. tomato paste

1 head of garlic (halved horizontally)

8 Tbsp. of butter

1 Tbsp. black peppercorns

2 sprigs of thyme

1 bay leaf

1 sprig of tarragon

1 bunch of parsley

2 cups of dry white wine

1 cup of Madeira wine

12 cups of water

1 gram sachet of cannabis

INSTRUCTIONS

In a larger stockpot, heat butter and a Tbsp. of olive oil. Add shells and let cook for 3–5 minutes, allowing butter to be fortified with the seafood flavor. Add onion, carrots, and garlic, and cook until onions are soft, stirring frequently. Add tomato paste, stir until vegetables and shells are coated. Add the herbs and peppercorns. Cook for 3 minutes. Deglaze with the white wine and reduce. Add the Madeira and cannabis, and cook for an additional 3–5 minutes. Add water and lower heat to simmer uncovered. Cook until it reduces by about half (8 cups). Strain into a freezer-safe container and use as needed.

You can substitute a ½ tsp. cannabis butter for the sachet of cannabis. (Yield slightly higher potency of 4.4 mg per cup of stock)

CAJUN STYLE BAYOU SHRIMP

YIELDS 2 SERVINGS AT 19.79 MG PER SERVING

2 Lbs. shrimp

2 Tbsp. garlic

2 Tbsp. roasted garlic and chive butter (reference recipe)

½ tsp. cannabis oil (reference recipe)

2 Tbsp. olive oil

½ tsp. cayenne pepper

1 tsp. scallions (chopped)

2 Tbsp. parsley

Pinch smoked paprika

1 tsp. house made lemon pepper (reference recipe)

4 Tbsp. white wine

1 tsp. garlic powder

½ tsp. white pepper

1 tsp. fresh thyme (chopped fine)

Kosher salt to taste

INSTRUCTIONS

In a large skillet, heat the cannabis oil and olive oil. Add shrimp and cook until opaque; add all seasonings and mix well. Deglaze with wine. Reduce on lower heat while stirring frequently. Slowly add chilled roasted garlic and chive butter and stir so that sauce emulsifies.

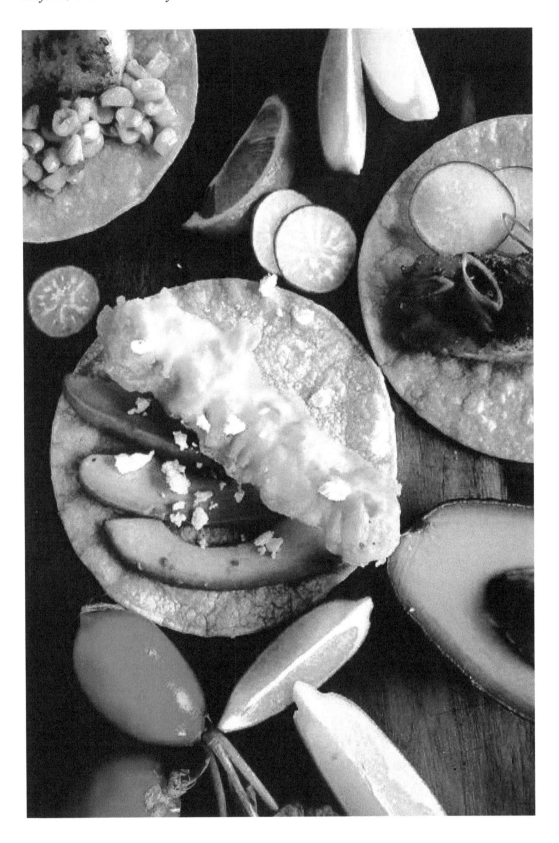

FRIED FISH TACOS

YIELDS 5 SERVINGS AT 2.25 MG AND

14.1MG PER SERVING (SERVED WITH CORN AND HERBED AIOLI)

5 2-ounce loins of Cod

¼ cup seltzer water

¼ cup Blue Moon Beer

½ cup all-purpose flour

Salt to taste

2 cups oil

INSTRUCTIONS

Whisk beer, seltzer water, flour, and salt. Heat oil (360 degrees). Coat fish in batter and fry in batches until golden (about 2 minutes). Drain on paper towel.

FRIED CORN INSTRUCTIONS

Take cleaned and shucked corn and rub it ferociously with garlic. Place the corn in aluminum foil and drizzle with olive oil; add split Thai chili and cilantro. Seal corn and bake at 350 degrees until tender.

Remove from oven and allow the corn to cool. Cut the corn off the cob and pat dry. Heat Chili Infused Cannabis Oil in a small skillet. Add the corn, salt to taste, and fry until slightly caramelized. Remove from heat, cool, and serve as condiment to tacos.

BLACKENED FISH TACOS

YIELDS 5 SERVINGS BETWEEN 8 AND 20 MG PER SERVING (SERVED WITH CORN AND HERBED AIOLI)

5 2-ounce loins of cod

5 Tbsp. blackened seasoning butter at room temp (reference recipe)

INSTRUCTIONS

Rub each loin with the appropriate amount of blackened seasoned cannabis butter. Heat cast-iron pan to a medium heat. Sear cod loins on each side for 2–3 minutes until cooked through.

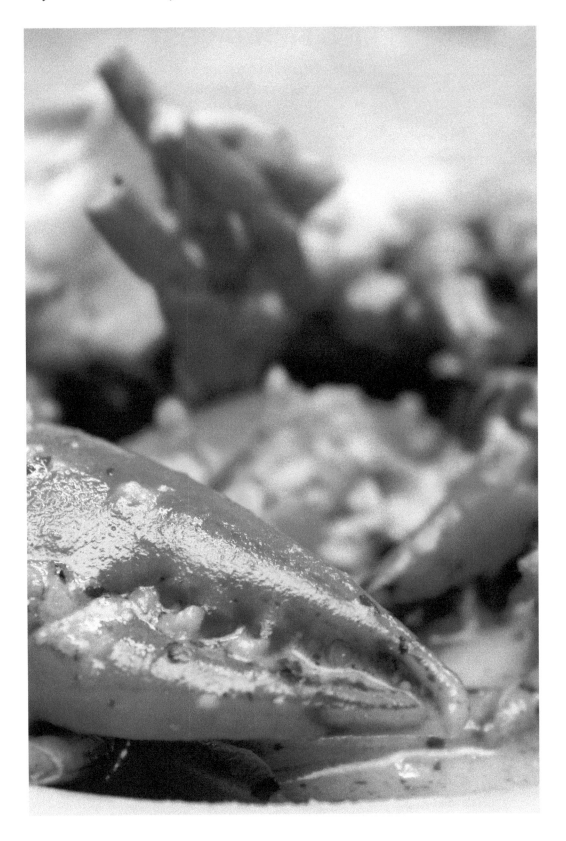

CRAB BOIL AND BISQUE STEW

YIELDS 4 SERVINGS AT 26.5 MG PER SERVING

8 red potatoes

8 Andouille sausages, sliced

1½ lbs. of pearl onions (cleaned)

2 ears fresh corn (halved)

2 cups dry white wine

½ cup Old Bay seasoning

4 whole crabs

12 large crawfish

4 large tiger shrimp (cleaned and deveined)

2 Tbsp. garlic powder

2 Tbsp. tomato paste

1 Tbsp. cumin

2 Tbsp. garlic (minced)

¼ cup onion (diced)

1 Thai Chili Pepper (minced fine)

*6 Roma tomatoes
(roasted, peeled, seeded, diced)*

8 cups of water

6 cups of seafood stock (reference recipe)

Heavy Cream

INGREDIENTS BROWN ROUX:

7½ Tbsp. butter

½ Tbsp. of clean cannabis butter

8 Tbsp. all-purpose flour

INSTRUCTIONS

Bring a Tbsp. of olive oil to medium heat and add corn, potatoes, and onions. Stir until onion becomes translucent; add seasonings, herbs, spices, and tomato paste and stir until ingredients are coated. Deglaze with wine. Add stock and water and cook down for 20 minutes. Add crabs, cook until done (3–5 minutes), and remove them. Add shrimp, cook until done (3–5 minutes), and remove them.

Add crawfish, cook until done (3–5 minutes), and remove them. Cook additionally until potatoes and corn are fork-tender, remove them. Reduce liquid down to 4 cups. Add tomatoes and roux; whisk until smooth. Add seafood, potatoes, and corn back to the pot with 2 ounces of heavy cream. Cook until mixture reaches desired soup consistency. Portion out in 4 equal servings and serve. Indulge with crusty bread.

ROUX:

Mix butter, cannabis butter, and flour until the roux is a golden brown color.

BUD PAIRING: For this I went with a pairing of XJ-13 for its citrus, pine, and earthy flavors. This dish represents everything about a good country boil that will leave you happy, euphoric, and uplifted. Additionally, the citrus notes balance well with the array of seafood, and the earthy notes compliment the red potatoes and sweet corn.

GARLIC CRABS

YIELDS 4 SERVINGS AT 14.MG PER SERVING

8 crabs, cleaned and cracked

1 whole bulb of garlic (finely chopped)

1 small onion (chopped)

1 cup butter (softened)

½ cup garlic cannabis butter (reference recipe)

½ tsp. salt

½ tsp. ground pepper

¼ tsp. red chili pepper flakes

INSTRUCTIONS

Place garlic, onions, butter, salt, and red and black pepper into a roasting pan, and put into a 450-degree oven.

Be sure to watch carefully and cook until onions and garlic turn golden brown.

Remove from oven, add crab, and blend thoroughly.

Make sure the crab (shells and all) is coated.

Place pan back into oven at 475 degrees for 15–20 minutes, turning crab about every 5 minutes.

After the crab has been heated throughout, remove from oven.

Garlic sauce should be braised onto the shell of the crab.

Serve as soon as possible, sprinkled with parsley and garnished with lemon.

ESCARGOT IN PUFF PASTRY

YIELDS 6 SERVINGS AT 23.5 MG PER SERVING

1 head garlic, separated into cloves (peeled and minced)

1 shallot (minced)

½ cup extra virgin olive oil

1 Tbsp. cannabis oil

½ cup butter

½ tsp. dried rosemary (finely chopped)

½ tsp. Thai (diced)

½ tsp. cumin

1 tsp. garlic powder

1 tsp. onion powder

¼ tsp. thyme

Salt and freshly ground black pepper

Parmesan cheese (sprinkle on top of puffs)

24 canned snails, drained and cut in half lengthwise

¼ cup Italian parsley (chopped)

1 sheet of frozen puff pastry, thawed

INSTRUCTIONS

Heat oil and butter. Add shallot and garlic and sauté 2 minutes. Add rosemary, thyme, and other spices. Simmer for 1 minute. Add snails and simmer for 30 minutes, stirring occasionally. Place 1 piece of snail in each of the 4 escargot bowl cups. Top with butter-garlic mixture. Cut out 24 1-inch rounds of puff pastry and top each snail with 1 round. Sprinkle Parmesan cheese on top. Bake at 400 degrees for 15–20 minutes, until pastry is puffed and lightly browned.

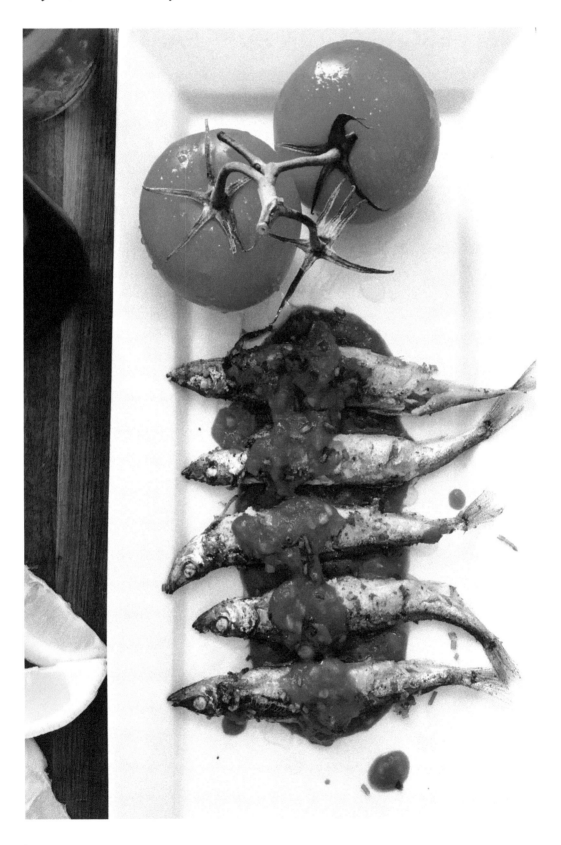

SARDINES IN TOMATO SAUCE

YIELDS 5 SERVINGS AT 18.8 MG PER SERVING

2 Tbsp., plus 3 Tbsp. olive oil

2 tsp. cannabis oil (reference recipe)

2 Tbsp. shallots, (minced)

4 cloves garlic (minced)

½ tsp. dried red pepper flakes

½ tsp. smoked paprika

1 Tbsp. tomato paste

½ cup white wine

¼ cup water

1 tsp. fish sauce

8–10 small fresh sardines
(cleaned and gutted)

2 tsp. salt

1 Tbsp. oregano (chopped)

½ tsp. thyme

1 tsp. umami paste

2 Tbsp. cilantro

INSTRUCTIONS

Heat the cannabis oil and 2 Tbsp. of the olive oil in a large ovenproof sauté pan over moderately high heat. Add the shallots, garlic, red pepper flakes, paprika, and umami paste and cook until the shallot becomes soft and translucent (3–5 minutes). Add the tomato paste and stir to combine, continuing to cook until the tomato paste just begins to brown.

Pour the wine into the pan and deglaze. Add the water and fish sauce and simmer until the liquid reduces and thickens. Remove from heat and set aside.

Season the sardines inside and out with the salt. Toss the sardines in the olive oil, making sure to coat inside and out.

Place sardines on top of tomato sauce and place in the oven. Cook until sardines have a crispy brown skin.

Serve with steamed rice.

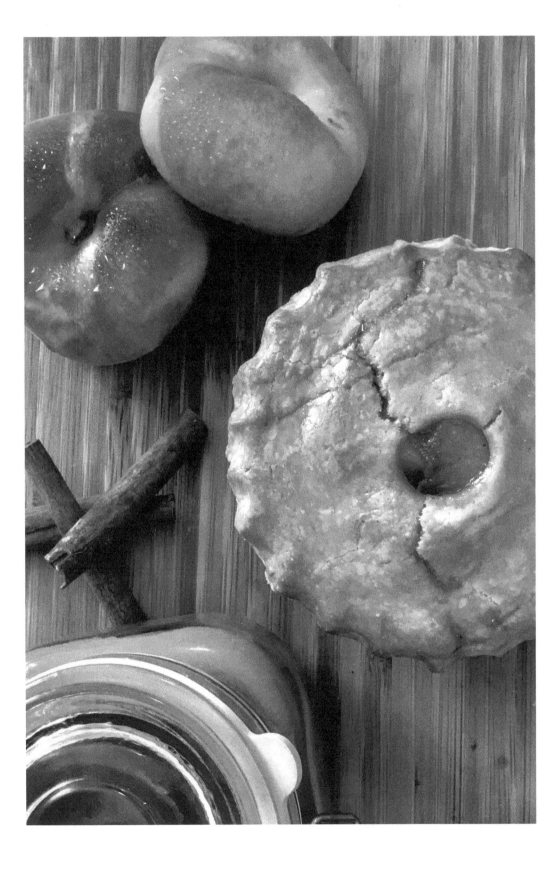

SWEETS AND TREATS

Growing up in my family, dessert was like the Westminster Dog Show; it only came around annually (at Thanksgiving) and was harshly critiqued by the judges, who in our case doubled as family members! Suffice to say, you had to bring your A game.

The consequence is that I was, and still am, not a great fan of desserts or sweets. I had the best of nature's sweets literally growing in my own back yard, what with the orange tree out back, the neighbor's tangerine tree next door, the mouth-watering tamarind tree one door down, and mango, pineapple, avocado, bananas, grapefruit, and Chinese plum trees on nearly every block. Not far from home, we would come across apple orchards, blueberry farms, peach groves, and scuppernongs! During non-harvest months we had the canned, preserved and pickled fruits and veggies we had prepared with leftovers!

But when the annual dog show came to town (i.e., Thanksgiving dinner), my mother and aunts would show up—dressed just shy of donning wide brim or pill top hats complete with lace veils, smiling broadly, with covered cake pans, fancy bakeware, and gleaming silver slicers.

They brought coffee cakes, caramel cakes, seven-up cakes, carrot cakes, and blueberry cakes; bread puddings, cobblers, cream puddings, and ambrosia; apple pie, pecan pie, sweet potato pie, and—the most dreaded—lemon meringue pie! Many of the aforementioned were on my list of 'avoid at all costs." If it didn't come with a fruit that was identifiable to the naked eye and there was no texture aside from the crust, I was never a fan.

However, there was guilt attached to my disdain of the family's dessert table. I wanted to like the wet mound of sweetened and baked day-old bread riddled with plump raisins. The rest of them thought it genius. And I tried for many consecutive years to eat a full slice of Grandma's glistening pecan pie! However, the high sugar content would send my taste buds into a quivering tailspin. Even now, the consideration of my dad's ambrosia makes me slightly nauseous.

I wanted to enjoy desserts as intently as my one aunt did. Her love of cakes and pies would have her sneaking into the kitchen when everyone else was engrossed in football or gearing up for round two. She'd hide away whole pies or massive portions of red velvet cake. Another aunt honored the desserts by piling a single plate with nearly every sugar packed option. I wanted to indulge in the chocolate cake and not discard it after two bites, but eventually I simply had to admit that I must not have inherited the sweet-loving dessert gene of my aunts.

Years later and as an adult, I learned that I could tell a different story. I could enjoy dessert as much as Cousin Shaun or Uncle Arthur. I was introduced to the perfect bite of pecan pie in Brooklyn, New York, of all places, on the very same stretch of Fulton Street where I found the Cake Man Raven and his award-winning red velvet cake. Though it took me two days to finish a single slice, I looked forward to every bite. I was reborn.

Though too much sugar can have detrimental effects, the solution does not have to be deprivation. Desserts can be reintroduced in a more inviting way. I redesigned bread pudding and redefined fruitcake. And, when I took my creations back home to those strictest of all judges, I found that they were welcome alternatives on the family table.

Lesson learned. In life, we do not have to accept others' truths as our own or abandon a concept. Break a few traditions and rules. Reinvent the wheel.

ROASTED CORN ICE CREAM

YIELDS 1.5 QUARTS (12 SCOOPS/SERVING) AT 17.5 MG PER SERVING

3 ears of corn

1 ¾ cup cannabis infused heavy cream (divided; reference recipe)

2 cups milk (separated)

1 cup granulated sugar (divided)

½ tsp. nutmeg

Pinch of salt

4 egg yolks

INSTRUCTIONS

Grill corn on medium-high heat for 10 minutes or until tender and slightly charred. Allow it to cool, cut kernels off the cob and place into a blender. Add 1 cup milk to the blender. Blend until pureed.

Place remaining ingredients except the egg yolks into a saucepan. Heat until it comes to a light simmer. Strain through a fine mesh strainer.

Beat eggs in a mixing bowl. Slowly pour the warm mixture into the eggs while continuing to beat the eggs until all of the mixture is incorporated. Transfer the mixture into a clean saucepan, and cook until the mixture has reached 180 degrees. Remove and let cool to room temperature before placing in the refrigerator to chill overnight.

Churn according to ice cream maker's instructions.

Place in the freezer for about 4 hours before serving. If eating after a day in the freezer, thaw it out a little to soften it up before scooping.

INFUSED HEAVY CREAM

YIELDS 4 CUPS AT 120 MG PER SERVING

4 cups heavy cream

2 grams cannabis in a sachet

INSTRUCTIONS

Place cream in saucepan with sachet and heat on very low temperature for 30 minutes. Allow to cool and squeeze sachet. Place cream in container and use as needed.

BREAD PUDDING

YIELDS 8 SERVINGS AT 6.7 MG PER SERVING

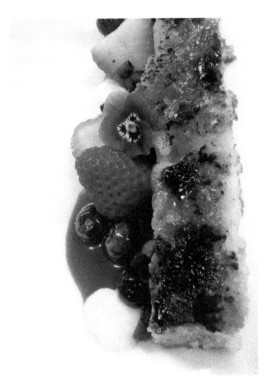

2 Tbsp. unsalted butter softened
(for baking dish)

½ Tbsp. clean cannabis butter
(reference recipe)

12 ounces brioche (cut into 1-inch cubes)

2 cups milk

3 cups heavy cream

4 large eggs (plus yolk of 1 large egg)

1 cup sugar

½ tsp. salt

1 Tbsp. pure vanilla extract

½ tsp. ground cinnamon

¼ tsp. ground nutmeg

1 cup boiling water (plus more for pan)

INSTRUCTIONS

Butter a 9x13-inch baking dish; set aside. Put bread in a large bowl; set aside. Heat cannabis, milk and cream in a medium saucepan over medium-high heat until just about to simmer; remove from heat.

Whisk eggs, yolk, sugar, salt, vanilla, cinnamon, and nutmeg in a medium bowl. Whisking constantly, pour cream mixture in a slow, steady stream into egg mixture. Pour over bread; fold to combine. Let stand 30 minutes, tossing and pressing occasionally to submerge bread.

Preheat oven to 350 degrees. With a slotted spoon, transfer bread to buttered dish; pour liquid in bowl over top. Using spoon, turn top layer of bread crust side up.

Set dish in a roasting pan, and transfer to oven. Pour boiling water into pan to reach about halfway up sides of dish. Bake until golden brown, about 50 minutes. Let dish cool on a rack for 10–20 minutes.

 BUD PAIRING: For this classic dessert, I chose a personal favorite, Blue Dream. This is great for its cerebral and invigorating properties, which makes it great for after-dinner conversations and creativity. I often serve this crowd favorite with seasonal berries, which complement the fruity notes of this strain.

FRUIT CAKE REIMAGINED

YIELDS 8 AT 14.1 MG PER SERVING

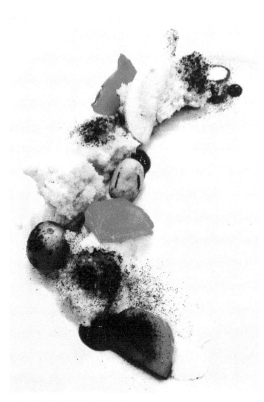

INSTRUCTIONS

Sift together a half cup of the sugar and 1 cup flour through a flour sifter or fine-mesh sieve into a bowl; set aside.

Note: be sure to use your largest mixing bowl for this next process—the mixture is going to have a lot of volume.

Make the Ener-G eggs in a large bowl (you'll need 6 Tbsp. of the powder whisked into 1 and a half cups warm water). Beat with a hand mixer for 12 minutes, until the mixture is thick and stiff like egg whites. After the first minute, add the cream of tartar and salt. At about the 6-minute mark, begin adding the remaining cup of sugar, 2 Tbsp. at a time.

Sift the cake flour mixture over the Ener-G mixture, a quarter cup at a time, and gently fold in. Fold in the vanilla extract.

Sift the remaining 2 Tbsp. cake flour. Spoon the batter into a 10-inch angel food cake pan, spreading evenly. Run a knife through the batter to break up any air pockets. Bake at 375 degrees for 40 minutes.

Remove from the oven and invert the pan over a plate.

Serve with charred grapes, basil and mint dust, ginger syrup glaze, and persimmons, lemon zest, and whipped coconut cream.

CAKE INGREDIENTS:

1 ½ cups vegan sugar, divided

1 cup cake flour

6 Tbsp. Ener-G egg replacer
(replaces 12 eggs)

1 ¼ tsp. cream of tartar

½ tsp. salt

1 tsp. vanilla extract

2 Tbsp. cake flour

Basil mint dust (reference recipe)

Coconut whipped cream (reference recipe)

BASIL MINT DUST

2 bunches of mint

2 bunches of basil

1 gram cannabis

INSTRUCTIONS

Heat oven to 150 degrees.

Place items on baking sheet in single
layer. Cook until all leaves dry.
Place in grinder and grind. Place in
airtight container and use as necessary.

COCONUT WHIP CREAM

*½ cup Let's Do...Organic Heavy
Coconut Cream*

1 tsp. baker's sugar

½ tsp. lemon zest

INSTRUCTIONS

Whip all ingredients.

BLOOD ORANGE SORBET

YIELDS 6 SERVINGS AT 20 MG PER SERVING

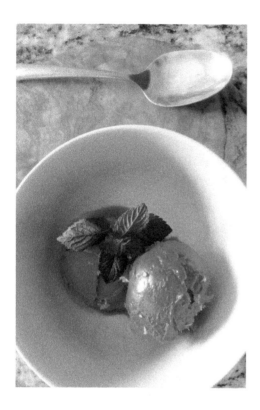

INSTRUCTIONS

To make the blood orange sorbet, combine the water, cannabis, and sugar in a small heavy-bottomed saucepan over medium heat. Bring just to a boil, whisking to dissolve the sugar. Remove the pan from the heat, remove sachet, and whisk in the blood orange juice and lemon juice. Pour the mixture into a shallow pan or bowl and refrigerate until completely chilled, 1 to 2 hours.

When the mixture is cold, pour it into an ice cream maker and process according to the manufacturer's instructions. If a soft sorbet is desired, serve immediately. If a firmer sorbet is desired, transfer the sorbet to an airtight glass or plastic freezer container, cover tightly, and freeze until firm, at least 4 hours.

¼ cup cold water

1 cup granulated sugar, or less to taste

2 cups blood orange juice, preferably freshly squeezed (from about 10 blood oranges)

1 Tbsp. lemon juice

¼ tsp. cardamom

½ gram cannabis sachet

FIVE-SPICE PEACH COBBLER

YIELDS 12 SERVINGS AT 18.1 MG PER SERVING

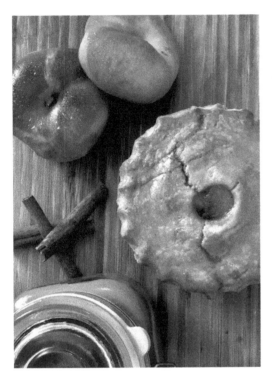

ELEVATED FIVE-SPICE SEASONING

YIELDS 11 SERVINGS (TSP.) AT 21 MG PER SERVING

2 Tbsp. dry star anise (ground)

2 Tbsp. fennel seed (ground)

2 tsp. cinnamon (ground)

2 tsp. Szechuan peppercorn (ground)

¼ tsp. cloves (ground)

1 tsp. cannabis (ground)

BUD PAIRING: For this, I went with the obvious choice but an elusive strain, Peaches and Cream. This wonderful bud has a sweet peachy flavor with citrus notes. This strain is great for focusing on tasks, should you need an extra push, or for unwinding after a long week.

28 ounces fresh sliced peaches (peeled)

1 cup sugar

1 tsp. cinnamon

Pinch of nutmeg

1 tsp. elevated five-spice seasoning 5.25 mg (reference recipe)

Pie crust (reference recipe)

INSTRUCTIONS

Combine peaches, sugar, and spices and place into pie crust laden ramekins. Place pie crust over ramekins. Bake 35–45 minutes at 350°F until golden brown.

PECAN TART

YIELDS 12 SERVINGS AT 17.6 MG PER SERVING

3½ cups coarsely chopped pecans

2 cups all-purpose flour

2/3 cup powdered sugar

12 Tbsp. butter (cubed)

½ cup firmly packed brown sugar

½ cup honey

2/3 cup butter

1 Tbsp. clean cannabis butter (reference recipe)

3 Tbsp. heavy cream

1 tsp. orange zest

1 ounce Grand Marnier

INSTRUCTIONS

Arrange pecans in a single layer on a baking sheet. Bake at 350° for 5–7 minutes or until lightly toasted. Cool on a wire rack 15 minutes or until completely cool.

Pulse flour, powdered sugar, and ¾ cup butter in a food processor 5 to 6 times or until mixture resembles coarse meal. Pat mixture evenly on bottom and sides of a lightly greased 4-inch tart/quiche pan with removable bottom.

Bake at 350° for 20 minutes or until edges are lightly browned. Cool on a wire rack 15 minutes or until completely cool.

Bring brown sugar, honey, ⅔ cup butter, cannabis butter, orange zest, grand Marnier, and whipping cream to a boil

in a 3-qt. saucepan over medium-high heat. Stir in toasted pecans, and spoon hot filling into prepared crust.

Bake at 350 degrees for 25–30 minutes or until golden and bubbly. Cool on a wire rack 30 minutes or until completely cool.

BUD PAIRING: This strain comes locked and loaded! Tangerine Dream is a hybrid of 3 strains, G13, Afghani, and Neville's A5 Haze. The earthiness of the pecans contrasts with the citrus orange, a sweet flavor providing the perfect balance for the Grand Marnier. This is a medical patient's favorite for its ability to knock out pain while leaving you energized (but too much will have you counting sheep).

CARAMEL APPLES

YIELDS 6 SERVINGS AT 14.1 MG PER SERVING

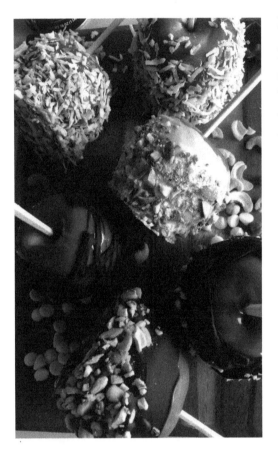

INSTRUCTIONS

Mix sugar, light corn syrup, and half cup of water in a small saucepan. Bring to a boil over medium-high heat, stirring just until the sugar dissolves. Cook, swirling the pan (do not stir) until the mixture is light amber and a candy thermometer registers 320 degrees, 8 to 10 minutes. Remove from the heat; slowly whisk in heavy cream, then butter, and then clean cannabis butter, vanilla extract, and a pinch of salt. Return to low heat and whisk until smooth. Let cool until the caramel is thick enough to coat a spoon. Insert sticks into the stem ends of 6 apples and dip the apples into the caramel, letting the excess drip off. Roll in toppings (tempered chocolate, coconuts, white baking chips, nuts, etc.) if desired, then let cool on a parchment-lined baking sheet coated with cooking spray.

6 Granny Smith apples

2 cups sugar

¼ cup light corn syrup

½ cup water

½ cup heavy cream

1 ½ Tbsp. cannabis butter (reference recipe)

½ Tbsp. butter

1 tsp. vanilla extract

Pinch of salt

COOKIES AND CREAM INFUSED FUDGE BITES

YIELDS 16 SERVINGS AT 26.5 MG PER SERVING

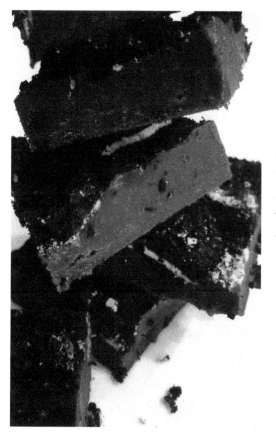

INSTRUCTIONS

Mix milk, butter, brown and granulated sugars, and salt in a heavy saucepan. Bring to a boil over medium heat, stirring constantly, for 6 minutes. Remove from heat and add vanilla paste, cocoa, and confectioner's sugar and beat with mixer until smooth and thick. Pour into prepped and buttered pan, press cookies into fudge, then freeze for 20 minutes. Unmold and cut into 16 1-ounce pieces. Enjoy!

½ cup cocoa

½ cup of milk

6 Tbsp. of clarified butter

2 Tbsp. clean cannabis butter (reference recipe)

½ cup brown sugar

½ cup granulated sugar

1 tsp. salt

1 tsp. vanilla bean paste

2 cups confectioner's sugar

1 cup of Oreo cookies (crushed)

BLACKBERRY DOOBIE

YIELDS 6 SERVINGS AT 17.5 MG PER SERVING

4 pints fresh blackberries

¾ cup sugar

1 tsp. grated ginger

½ cup water

3 ½ Tbsp. butter

*½ Tbsp. clean cannabis butter
(reference recipe)*

2 Tbsp. cornstarch dissolved in ¼ cup water

2 cup self-rising flour

2 Tbsp. sugar

½ cup vegetable shortening

2/3 cup milk

Raw sugar (for rolling dumpling balls on)

INSTRUCTIONS

Heat oven to 350 degrees.

In a deep 12-inch skillet, toss the berries,
sugar, water ginger, and butter.
Bring to a simmer over medium heat,
stirring often. Reduce the heat to low
and simmer for 5 minutes. Stir in the
dissolved cornstarch and cook until the
juices thicken, about 1 minute.

Meanwhile, make the dumplings: In a
medium bowl, mix the flour and sugar.
Add the shortening. Using a fork or a
pastry blender, cut the shortening into the
flour until the mixture resembles coarse
crumbs. Using a fork, stir in the milk.
Roll dumpling dough into balls.

Place blackberry doobie filling into
ramekins. Drop the dumplings in each
ramekin. Place ramekins in water bath
and place in oven until golden brown.
Serve hot.

Garnish with toasted almond pieces.

As I've often said, I prefer savory foods
to sweets, but there is one exception: my
mother's teacakes.

TEA CAKES

YIELDS 8 SERVINGS AT 14.1 MG PER SERVING

The beauty of these gems is that they aren't excessively sweet. Initially, their versatility escaped me, but now I have learned that they can be paired magnificently with fresh fruit, preserves, cheeses, hams, and honeys.

As a monthly treat, my mother would whip up a cool batch of her warm teacakes, usually on a Saturday evening as my siblings and I crowded around the television to take in a special feature of *The Blob*, *Godzilla*, *The Birds*, or *The Shining*. The movie was inconsequential to me, as I was the youngest of my siblings and never had a say in the selection anyway. My sole interest was in the smell of mom's warm teacakes.

The faint aroma of the sweetened bread would waft through the house and I would anxiously inquire, "Are they ready yet?" I would always get shooed from the kitchen after a third or fourth check-in.

Finally, after what seemed like an eternity, mom would plate the cake-like cookies and plop them in front of us. Slowly and deliberately, I would break open the warm teacake, savoring it bite after bite. I would identify to myself the various flavors—vanilla, lemon, almond extract, or nutmeg (depending on what was in the cupboard). I made mental notes for myself of the lightness and the mild sugary flavor that was perfection for my youthful palate. By the time the special

feature ended and my siblings were wide-awake and ready for cakes, I was off to a sound teacake dreamland slumber, full as a tick.

1 cup butter

1¾ cups white sugar

2 eggs

3 cups all-purpose flour

½ tsp. baking soda

½ tsp. salt

¼ tsp. ground nutmeg

1 tsp. vanilla extract

INSTRUCTIONS

In a medium bowl, cream together the butter and sugar until smooth. Beat in the eggs one at a time, then stir in the vanilla. Combine the flour, baking soda, salt and nutmeg; stir into the creamed mixture. Knead dough for a few times on a floured board until smooth. Cover and refrigerate until firm.

Preheat the oven to 325 degrees F (165 degrees C). On a lightly floured surface, roll the dough out to 1/4 inch in thickness. Cut into desired shapes with cookie cutters. Place cookies 1 1/2 inches apart onto cookie sheets.

Bake for 8 to 10 minutes in the preheated oven. Allow cookies to cool on baking sheet for 5 minutes before removing to a wire rack to cool completely.

SWEET TEA CRÈME BRÛLÉE

YIELDS 8 SERVINGS AT 15 MG PER SERVING

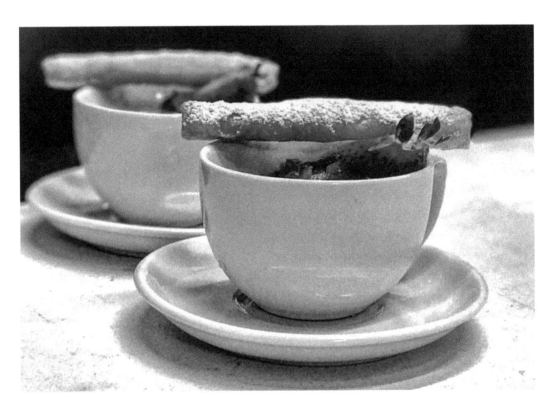

1 cup infused heavy cream
(reference recipe)

3 cups heavy cream

¾ cups sugar

1 vanilla bean, split lengthwise

7 large egg yolks

¼ tsp. kosher salt

2 Lipton tea bags

INSTRUCTIONS

Prepare oven and baking dishes: Heat oven to 300 degrees. Bring a kettle or pot of water to a boil. Place 8 5-ounce baking dishes in a large roasting pan.

Gently heat cream: In a medium saucepan, combine cream and half the sugar (¼ cup plus 2 Tbsp.). Scrape vanilla bean seeds into pan, then add pod. Add tea bags. Heat over medium heat just until mixture starts to bubble around the edge of the pan, 7–8 minutes, making sure it doesn't boil. Remove tea bags.

Meanwhile, whisk the egg yolks in a large mixing bowl with salt and remaining sugar.

Temper eggs: Use ladle to pour a small amount of the hot cream mixture into the egg mixture, and then whisk to combine, making sure to prevent the eggs from curdling. Add 2 more ladles of cream mixture, one at a time, whisking to combine after each addition. Gradually whisk in remaining cream mixture. Strain through a fine sieve into a large liquid measuring cup (to remove the vanilla pod and any bits of cooked egg).

Bake: Divide custard evenly among baking dishes. Place pan in oven. Add enough boiling water to come halfway up the sides of the dishes. Bake until custards are just set, about 30–40 minutes.

Chill: Remove pan from oven. Use tongs to carefully remove dishes from hot-water bath and place on a wire rack for 30 minutes. Then, cover with plastic wrap and chill for at least 2 hours (or up to 3 days) before serving. The custard will finish setting in the refrigerator.

Caramelize tops and serve: Sprinkle raw sugar over each custard. Working with one at a time, pass the flame of the torch in a circular motion 1 to 2 inches above the surface of each custard until the sugar bubbles, turns amber, and forms a smooth surface. Serve immediately.

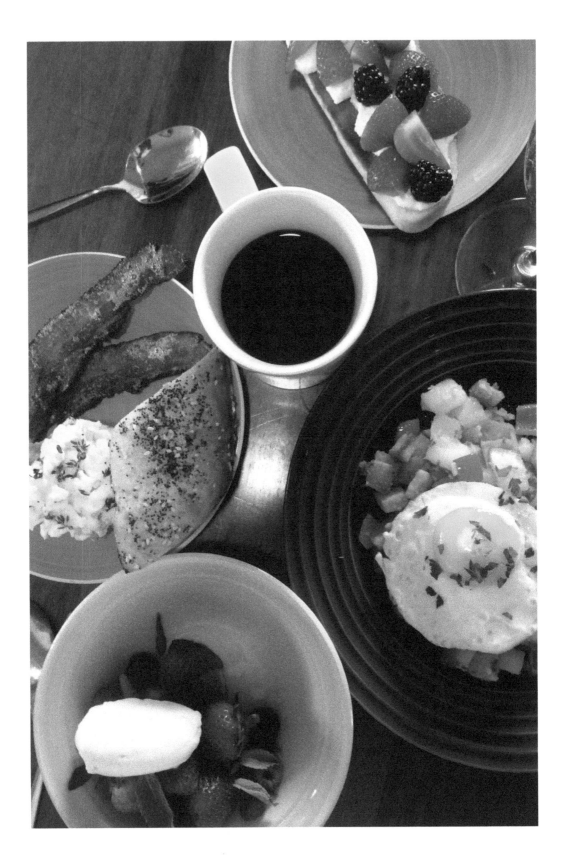

THE BUSINESS OF BRUNCH

I never quite understood why we needed to designate particular foods for breakfast, lunch, or dinner. It seemed to me that if food was sourced properly, was healthy, and was desired, any category of food should be fair game for any meal. Nowadays, seeing how many Americans eat cereal for dinner, I can see that I am not alone in this belief. Why must we have eggs for breakfast, sandwiches for lunch, and a heavy protein and starch meal for dinner? I would propose eggs and leftover fried chicken for breakfast, or jellied toast and fried deli meat (classic). I always loved and craved the interplay of sweet and savory.

Imagine my delight when I discovered brunch! I had to grow up first. I had to leave home. I had to reach the legal drinking age. It's not that I hadn't had a meal of similar components at the appropriate brunch time of day. It's just that I hadn't had it formally, with a fancy name attached and cocktail offerings on the opposite side of the menu. In no time, this officially became my favorite meal of all time.

SHRIMP AND POPCORN GRITS

YIELDS 4 SERVINGS AT 35.25 MG PER SERVING

INGREDIENTS FOR SHRIMP:

12 large Australian prawns or tiger shrimp (cleaned and deveined)

8 mussels (cleaned and debearded)

1 cup shrimp stock

⅛ cup oil

⅛ cup butter

¼ Tbsp. clean cannabis butter (reference recipe)

½ cup dry white wine

¼ cup flour, plus extra flour as needed to form a paste

½ okra (cut on the bias)

¼ cup green bell pepper (chopped)

1½ garlic cloves (minced)

½ tsp. cayenne pepper or to taste

2 cups seafood stock

Kosher salt to taste

½ cup minced green onions, plus extra for garnish

½ cup of bacon or pork belly (cooked crispy for garnish)

INGREDIENTS FOR POPCORN GRITS

¼ cup popcorn kernels

1 cup stone ground grits (cooked)

½ tsp. clean cannabis butter (reference recipe)

2 Tbsp. butter

2 cups water plus more as needed

Salt to taste

INSTRUCTIONS FOR SHRIMP:

Heat a couple Tbsp. of oil to close to the smoke point in a medium skillet; add okra and pan sear until it reaches mild caramelization. Remove from skillet and set aside.

Lower heat on oil. Salt prawns and add to skillet. Cook until opaque (halfway through). Remove from skillet and set aside.

Add wine to small saucepan, bring to a medium boil, and add cleaned mussels. Salt lightly and cover. Cook until the mussels open and remove from heat immediately.

To make the roux, melt butter (including cannabis butter) with oil in a large heavy saucepan over low heat. Whisk flour into the oil to form a paste while cooking over low heat and whisking continuously until the mixture turns a caramel color and gives off a nutty aroma, about 15–20 minutes.

Add the green pepper and garlic, and cook over low heat until the vegetables are limp, about 5 minutes.

Add the cayenne pepper, seafood stock, and salt to taste. Bring to a boil, reduce the heat to low, and simmer for 10 to 15 minutes until mixture thickens.

Add shrimp and simmer until shrimp is cooked through. Remove from heat and add the drained mussels.

INSTRUCTIONS FOR POPCORN GRITS:

In a large stockpot, bring a generous amount of vegetable oil to smoking. Add a layer of popcorn kernels and cover. Move the pot and keep it in motion until kernels began to pop.

Note: Moving the pot helps to evenly distribute the heat so that the kernels do not burn.

Lower the heat to medium-high while continuing to move the pot until the popping lessens. Uncover and pour kernels into a bowl. Remove any darkened or charred kernels.

Place 2 cups of water, 2 Tbsp. of butter, and salt to taste in a separate saucepan and bring to a simmer. Add a generous handful of popcorn and cook until softened (30 seconds to 1 minute). Strain the wet kernels through a fine mesh sieve, and discard hulls and seeds. Add more popcorn to the simmering liquid and repeat the process until you've rendered 3 complete cups of popcorn mush (grits). Add more water if needed.

Transfer the strained popcorn mush, which will look like stiff grits, into a pot with 1 cup of cooked stone ground grits. Add the reserved cooking liquid, which should be slightly thickened from the cornstarch and should taste like popcorn.

Add butter and more water as necessary to create desired thickness and texture.

Plate 1 cup of grits per serving. Add 3 prawns and 2 mussels per plate. Finish with equal parts etouffee sauce, and garnish with seared okra, bacon, and green onion.

CRABCAKES BENEDICT

YIELDS 4 SERVINGS AT 15.5 MG PER SERVING

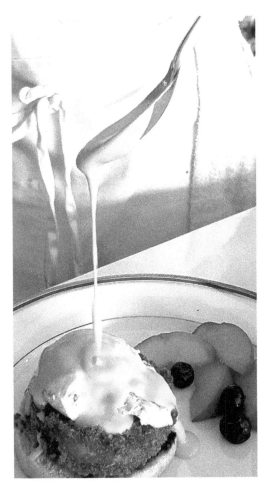

INGREDIENTS FOR CRAB CAKES:

1 lb. jumbo lump crabmeat

1 Tbsp. tarragon (minced)

1 Tbsp. parsley (minced)

2 cloves garlic (minced)

1 tsp. garlic powder

1 Tbsp. Dijon mustard

2 Tbsp. of infused mayonnaise (reference recipe)

½ tsp. cayenne pepper

Kosher salt to taste

1 large egg

2 cups panko

Canola oil

2 toasted English muffins

INGREDIENTS FOR HOLLANDAISE SAUCE:

YIELDS 6 SERVINGS AT 11.6 MG PER SERVING

½ cup clarified butter

1 tsp. clean cannabis butter (reference recipe)

3 egg yolks

2 tsp. lemon juice

½ tsp.cayenne pepper

½ tsp. Dijon mustard

Kosher salt to taste

INSTRUCTIONS

CRAB CAKES

Put the jumbo lump crab into a mixing bowl. Add in the tarragon, garlic, mustard, garlic powder, cayenne, infused mayonnaise, 1 beaten egg, and parsley. Mix well. Season the crab mixture with salt.

Form the crab into 6 2½-ounce patties. Press each crab cake in panko breadcrumbs. Place them onto a small baking sheet and chill in the refrigerator for about 30 minutes before cooking.

Heat oil to 350 degrees. Deep fry crab cakes until golden.

HOLLANDAISE (1½ CUPS)

Melt the butter in a small saucepan over low heat. Place the egg yolks, cayenne, mustard, and lemon juice into a blender. Blend until the mixture is foamy and slightly stiffened.

With the blender running, gradually add the clarified butter in a thin stream. Season to taste with kosher salt.

The sauce should be served within an hour. Keep in a warm spot.

POACHED EGGS

Heat a pot of water to a bare simmer. Crack an egg into a small bowl or ramekin, and gently slip the egg into the water. Do this for each egg. Turn off the heat, cover the pot, and let sit for 4 minutes or until egg whites are solid. Gently remove eggs with slotted spoon. Place on top of toasted English muffin, spoon hollandaise over the egg; serve with your favorite cocktail.

 BUD PAIRING: The Sage strain has earthy spicy, and pine undertones, and it's great for pain relief, leaving you in a happy, relaxed, uplifted mood.

STUFFED FRENCH TOAST

YIELDS 8 SERVINGS AT 27 MG PER SERVING

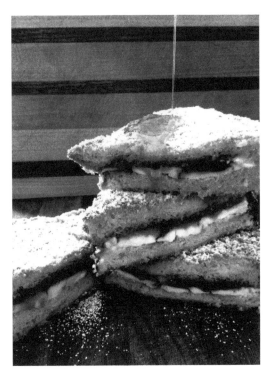

1 loaf brioche bread

8 ounces cream cheese (soft)

¼ cup raspberry jam (reference recipe)

½ tsp. orange zest

*½ cup fresh raspberries
(plus more for garnish)*

1 cup whole milk

*1 Tbsp. clean cannabis butter
(melted; reference recipe)*

2 Tbsp. butter (not melted)

1 Tbsp. brown sugar

2 tsp. vanilla extract

1½ tsp. ground cinnamon

3 large eggs

Powdered sugar (garnish)

Maple syrup (for serving)

INSTRUCTIONS

In a small mixing bowl, combine fresh raspberries (mashed), raspberry jam, and orange zest.

In a baking dish, whisk together the milk, 1 Tbsp. melted cannabis butter, brown sugar, vanilla, cinnamon, and eggs.

In a large, heavy-bottomed skillet melt the 2 Tbsp. butter over medium heat.

Spread raspberry mixture on 1 slice of bread; spread cream cheese on other slice of bread and close to make a sandwich. Once the slices are "stuffed," place each combined double slice into the milk and egg mixture for about 10 seconds per side. Once the slices are coated, place them into the skillet to brown. Work in batches. Cook each slice of stuffed French toast until golden brown.

Keep cooked French toast on baking sheet in 200-degree oven to keep warm as you make the rest of the French toast. Serve warm, topped with extra berries, powdered sugar, and maple syrup.

BUTTERMILK BISCUITS AND RED EYE SAUSAGE GRAVY

YIELDS 12 SERVINGS AT 23.4 MG PER SERVING

1 lb. coarsely ground pork

¼ cup onion (chopped fine)

2 garlic cloves (minced)

1 tsp. brown sugar

1½ tsp. ground sage

¾ tsp. salt

½ tsp. parsley (minced)

Pinch of nutmeg

2 tsp. fennel seed

¼ tsp. pepper flakes

1 Tbsp. cooking oil

1 Tbsp. ground pork fat

2 tsp. packed brown sugar

¾ cup strong black coffee

1 tsp. clean cannabis butter (reference recipe)

Biscuits (reference recipe)

BUTTERMILK BISCUITS:

1¼ cup bread flour

1¼ cup pastry flour

13 Tbsp. butter

1 Tbsp. clean cannabis butter (reference recipe)

1¼ Tbsp. baking powder

2 Tbsp. sugar

13 ounces buttermilk

2½ tsp. salt

INSTRUCTIONS

In a medium bowl combine the pork, onion, garlic, the tsp. of brown sugar, sage, salt, parsley, nutmeg, fennel, and pepper flakes. Mix thoroughly. Shape mixture into twelve 3-inch patties using wet hands. Arrange on a tray. Cover; refrigerate overnight.

In a large skillet, fry patties, half at a time, in hot oil over medium heat for 5 minutes on each side, or until browned and cooked through. Remove from heat: keep warm.

For the Red-Eye Gravy, stir the 2 Tbsp. brown sugar into the drippings in the skillet, then add the tsp. of cannabis butter. Stir in the coffee. Bring to a boil. Boil gently, uncovered, for 2 or 3 minutes or until gravy is slightly thickened and has a rich reddish-brown color.

BISCUIT INSTRUCTIONS

Sift dry ingredients into a bowl. Break up the butter into the dry ingredients. Mix in mixing bowl until it resembles coarse cornmeal. Add liquid ingredients. Mix liquid ingredients with dry and combine. Knead lightly. Roll out the dough onto a floured surface. Use round or square cookie cutter to portion out 12 servings. Place each biscuit on cooking sheet. Bake at 375 degrees until biscuits are slightly golden.

PANZANELLA HASH SALAD WITH A SUNNY SIDE UP EGG

YIELDS 8 AT 17.6 MG PER SERVING

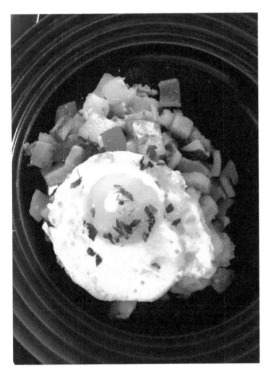

1 small loaf Italian bread (cut into 1-inch thick slices)

3 Tbsp. olive oil (divided)

8 ounces heirloom cherry tomatoes

¼ tsp. kosher salt

1 cup potato (diced and cooked)

1 cup crispy prosciutto

12 ounces fresh bocconcini balls

4 Tbsp. grated parmesan cheese

8 sunny side up eggs

DRESSING:

1 Thai chili pepper

4 cloves garlic

1 bunch cilantro (cleaned and stemmed)

1½ bunches basil (cleaned and stemmed)

½ bunch mint (cleaned and stemmed)

3 anchovies

2 Tbsp. nutritional yeast flakes

1 Tbsp. Dijon mustard

½ lemon (juice)

1/8 cup champagne vinegar

½ cup water

1 Tbsp. cannabis oil (reference recipe)

¾ cup olive oil

INSTRUCTIONS

In a blender, add Thai pepper, garlic, cilantro, basil, mint, anchovies, yeast flakes, Dijon mustard, lemon juice, vinegar, and water. Blend until loose (add water if needed). Turn blender on low and puree. Add oil in a slow stream until all ingredients come together. My preference is medium thickness, like a Caesar dressing. However, you can add more lemon juice or water to obtain the thickness that you desire. Salt to taste.

Preheat oven to 350 degrees.

Drizzle bread with olive oil and season with salt and pepper. Place in the oven and cook until golden and toasted. Remove from oven and cool.

On a separate baking sheet, place the tomatoes in a single layer, drizzle with oil, salt to taste, and bake until slightly blistered. Remove from oven and cool.

In a small skillet, bring 3 Tbsp. of vegetable oil to medium-high heat, then add boiled diced potatoes. Fry until golden. Remove and cool.

In a large mixing bowl, combine 2½ cups bread, bocconcini, cherry tomatoes, salt and pepper, potatoes, crispy prosciutto, and dressing, then toss to evenly coat.

Evenly apportion 8 servings

BUD PAIRING: Trinity is a rare sativa strain that was selected for its earthy, flowery, and lemon undertones. This pairing will leave you euphoric, relaxed, and energized so you can easily get through that to-do list.

SUNNY SIDE UP EGGS

Ingredients:
4 tsp. olive oil
8 large eggs
Kosher salt to taste

INSTRUCTIONS

On low heat, heat the oil in a pan in medium nonstick pan. Gently crack egg into pan (no more than 3 eggs at a time) so that you do not overcrowd the pan. Cover with a clear lid and cook until the whites are completely set but the yolks are still runny (about 2 minutes). Gently remove from pan, being careful not to break yolk and serve.

PEACHY KEEN COCKTAIL

YIELDS 8 SERVINGS AT 13.75 MG PER SERVING

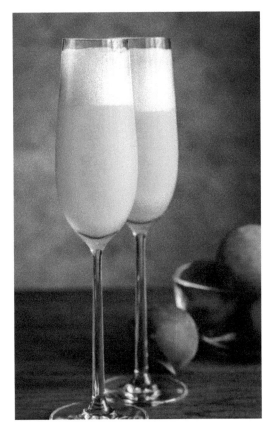

8 ounces (1 cup) ginger peach puree (reference recipe)

Bottle of Prosecco*

INSTRUCTIONS

Portion 1 ounce of puree for each champagne flute (8 total), and top off with Prosecco. Stir and garnish with strawberries.

* A good ginger ale can be substituted for the champagne.

CARAMELIZED ONION FRITTATA BLISTERED TOMATOES & GARGONZOLA

YIELDS 2 SERVINGS AT 7.5 MG PER SERVING

2 Tbsp. garlic roasted cannabis oil (reference recipe)

¼ cup caramelized onion

4 eggs (whisked)

1 tsp. kosher salt

¼ cup crème fraîche

1 cup plum tomatoes

2 Tbsp. Gorgonzola cheese

1 tsp. lemon juice

1 Tbsp. water

3 Tbsp. buttermilk

Parsley for garnish

INSTRUCTIONS

Preheat the oven to 400 degrees.

Drizzle tomatoes with olive oil and season lightly with kosher salt. Place tomatoes on baking sheet in a single layer, and then bake in oven until tomatoes blister (5–10 minutes). Set aside for garnish.

Blend crème fraîche with lemon juice and Gorgonzola, and set aside for garnish.

Whisk eggs with 3 Tbsp. of buttermilk and 1 Tbsp. of water. Salt to taste.

Evenly spread caramelized onions in small cast-iron skillet. Pour eggs over the onions. Cook for 1 minute, and then place the pan in the oven and cook 6 minutes or until eggs are cooked. Top with tomatoes, cheese blend, and parsley and serve.

VINYL (THE OFFICIAL ELEVATION COCKTAIL)

YIELDS 16 SERVINGS AT 15 MG PER SERVING

INGREDIENTS FOR SIMPLE SYRUP:

2 cups sugar

2 cups water

1 cup lemon zest

¼ cup lemon juice

1½ large ancho chilies (dried and seeded)

½ tsp. liquid smoke

1 gram ground cannabis sachet

INSTRUCTIONS

Add sugar to medium saucepan. Bring to a medium heat and add water, lemon zest, lemon juice, and cannabis. Toast ancho chilies over an open flame, and then add to the pot. Reduce by a quarter of a cup. Add liquid smoke. Stir. Remove from heat and cool.

COCKTAIL INSTRUCTIONS

Pour 1 ounce simple syrup and 1½ ounce mescal over large ice cube and stir. Garnish with lemon peel and smoked jerky.

BUD PAIRING: This strain comes locked and loaded! Tangerine Dream is a hybrid of three strains, G13, Afghani, and Neville's A5 Haze. I paired this to contrast the earthiness of the pecans with a citrus, orange, sweet flavor providing the perfect balance for the Grand Marnier. This is a medical patient's favorite for its ability to knock out pain while leaving you energized (but too much will have you counting sheep).

SOFT SCRAMBLED EGGS WITH SAUTÉED BROCCOLINI

YIELDS 4 SERVINGS AT 22.5 MG PER SERVING

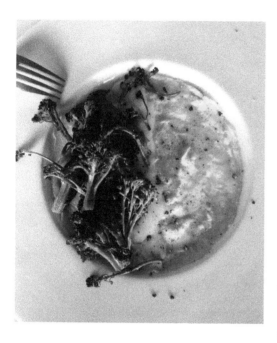

INSTRUCTIONS

Beat eggs, buttermilk, and water until combined.

In a medium-sized skillet, add the garlic roasted cannabis oil and bring to a medium heat, then add garlic and sauté until soft. Add broccolini and chili flakes. Salt to taste. Cook until broccolini is al dente.

Bring separate skillet to medium-high heat. Add a half Tbsp. of butter and 1 Tbsp. of oil to the skillet, add egg mixture, and move gently with rubber spatula until scrambled soft.

Portion evenly onto serving plates and add 1 ounce of Brie per plate. To set, place into low temperature oven for 30 seconds to 1 minute. Serve with garlic broccolini. Garnish with fresh cracked pepper.

8 eggs

2 ounces of infused buttermilk (reference recipe)

1 ounce water

Kosher salt to taste

1 lb. broccolini

2 cloves garlic (minced fine)

1 Tbsp. garlic roasted cannabis oil (reference recipe)

1/8 tsp. chili flakes

½ Tbsp. butter

4 ounces diced Brie

RICOTTA PANCAKES

YIELDS 6 SERVINGS AT 9.6 MG PER SERVING

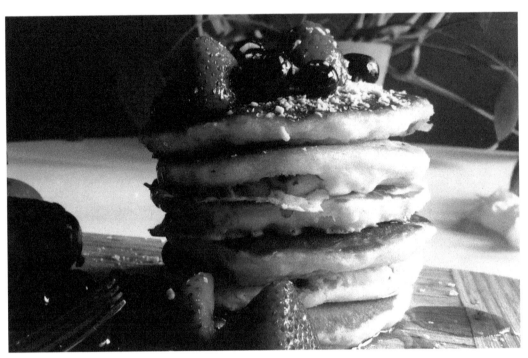

⅔ cup of all-purpose flour

⅓ cup baker's sugar

½ tsp. baking powder

¼ tsp. baking soda

¼ tsp. kosher salt

¾ cup ricotta cheese (drained)

3 eggs (separated)

1 tsp. vanilla bean paste

¼ cup infused buttermilk

2 Tbsp. water

Homemade syrup (reference recipe)

INSTRUCTIONS

In a large mixing bowl, combine the dry ingredients: flour, baking powder, baking soda, sugar, and salt. Mix well. In a separate bowl combine ricotta, egg yolks, vanilla bean paste, infused buttermilk, and water. Add to flour mixture and stir until smooth.

In a clean bowl, beat egg whites until stiff peaks form. Using rubber spatula, gently fold a quarter of beaten egg whites into ricotta mixture. Then gently fold in the rest of the beaten egg whites.

For each pancake, scoop a quarter cup batter onto oiled non-stick skillet. Turn when bubbles form at the top of each pancake and edges are golden. Serve with 1 ounce of homemade syrup.

BRÛLÉED APRICOTS WITH BLACKBERRY AND CHANTILLY CREAM

YIELDS 4 SERVINGS AT 15 MG PER SERVING

½ cup infused cream (reference recipe)

2 tsp. of baker's sugar

1 tsp. lemon zest

6 apricots (pitted and halved)

1 cup turbinado sugar

1 cup of blackberries (or other seasonal berries)

2 Tbsp. homemade maple syrup (reference recipe)

INSTRUCTIONS

Preheat oven to 300 degrees.

Place apricots on a small baking sheet and heat in the oven until slightly softened. Remove and set aside to cool.

In a small chilled mixing bowl, add cream and baker's sugar. Whisk to soft peaks. Incorporate lemon zest thoroughly.

Coat each apricot half in turbinado sugar. Use kitchen torch to brûlée each half. Coat blackberries with homemade maple syrup.

Place 3 halves of apricot, ¼ cup of berries, and equal portions of cream on plate.

Serve and enjoy.

SHAKSHUKA FUSION

YIELDS 6 SERVINGS AT 11.6 MG TPER SERVING

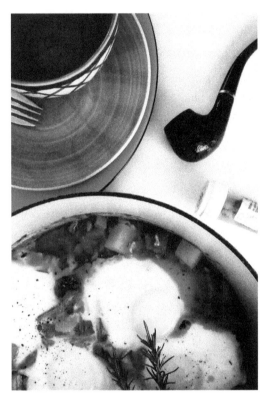

1/4 cup olive oil

1 tsp. cannabis oil (reference recipe)

1 tube soy chorizo
(preferably Trader Joe's brand)

2 Thai chili peppers

1 small yellow onion (chopped)

5 cloves of garlic (minced)

1 tsp. ground cumin

1/2 Tbsp. paprika

1/2 Tbsp. smoked paprika

1 can of diced tomatoes
(28 ounces undrained)

Kosher salt to taste.

1/2 cup diced potatoes (cooked al dente)

1 tsp. of rosemary (chopped fine)

1/2 Tbsp. tomato powder (tomato paste can
be substituted for tomato powder)

Crusty bread for serving

INSTRUCTIONS

In a large saucepot, heat oil on medium-high heat. Add chopped chili peppers and onions; cook until soft and slightly golden. Add cumin, paprika, smoked paprika, and garlic, and cook for 1 minute. Add the rosemary and chorizo. Cook until chorizo is firm. Stir frequently.

Add diced tomatoes (and liquid), along with half cup of water and tomato powder. Reduce heat to medium, simmer, and stir occasionally until slightly thickened.

Crack eggs over the sauce and cover. Cook until whites are cooked through and the yolks are set.

Serve with crusty bread.

BUD PAIRING: It seems befitting to use a strain called Outlaw in this era of cannabis prohibition. The spicy and herbaceous notes of this sativa were a slam-dunk in pairing with this North African inspired dish. The earthy flavor of this pepped-up strain is perfect with the cumin, smoked paprika, and spicy chorizo.

KIMCHI FRIED RICE

YIELDS 2 SERVINGS AT 27.3 MG PER SERVING

1 Tbsp. vegetable oil

1 tsp. cannabis oil (reference recipe)

1 Tbsp. of garlic roasted cannabis oil (to drizzle; reference recipe)

½ cup chopped chicken, beef, or tofu

3 cups day-old short grain rice

3 finely sliced scallions (without whites)

1 cup kimchi (roughly chopped)

Kimchi juice (as needed)

2 tsp. toasted sesame oil

1 tsp. soy sauce

2 eggs

Sesame seeds (for garnish)

INSTRUCTIONS

Heat oil and cannabis oil in a wok or a large skillet over medium-high heat. Add meat and cook, stirring occasionally, until cooked through (about 2–3 minutes). Meanwhile, place rice in a large bowl, and drizzle with the garlic roasted cannabis oil. With your hands, separate rice grains as much as possible without smashing or breaking them. Use just enough oil to coat each grain.

Add the white parts of the scallions to the pan and cook just until fragrant, about 30 seconds. Add the kimchi and juice and stir to toss. Add the rice and toss to coat, distributing the ingredients evenly. Allow the rice to cook for about 10 minutes, tossing halfway through, or as needed to keep the bottom of the rice from burning.

Drizzle with the sesame oil and soy sauce, and toss to distribute evenly. Cook for another 3–5 minutes, tossing as needed to keep the bottom of the rice from burning. Taste for seasoning, and add a sprinkling more sesame oil and soy sauce, if desired. Reserve a handful of green onions, and toss the rest in the pan with the rice. Quickly give it a toss to distribute, and then divide rice between 2 bowls.

In a small pan, fry both eggs and use to top the kimchi fried rice. Garnish with reserved green onions and sesame seeds.

ELEVATED HOT CHOCOLATE

YIELDS 4 SERVINGS AT 15 MG PER

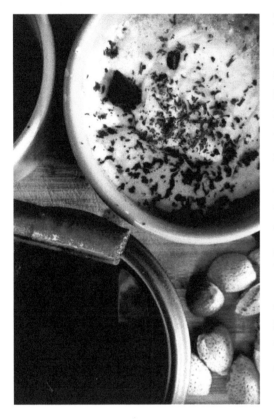

INSTRUCTIONS

Combine the cocoa and sugar in a saucepan. Add boiling water, and bring this mixture to an easy boil while stirring. Slowly add the chocolate chips and stir until melted. Simmer and stir for about 2 minutes.

Stir in 3½ cups of milk and heat until very hot, but do not allow the mixture to come to a boil. Remove from heat, and add vanilla or other flavor. Divide between 4 mugs.

Add 2 Tbsp. of infused cream to each mug. Add 1 ounce of Frangelico or Chambord to each mug (optional). Stir and serve.

⅓ cup unsweetened cocoa powder

¾ cup white sugar

1 cup Ghirardelli chocolate chip morsels

⅓ cup boiling water

3 ½ cups milk

¾ tsp. vanilla extract

½ cup infused cream

4 ounces Frangelico or Chambord (optional)

HOMEMADE PEANUT BUTTER SERVED WITH BRÛLÉED BANANAS

YIELDS 3 CUPS AT 4.2 MG THC PER 1 TBSP. SERVING

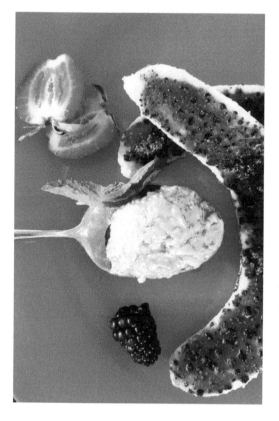

INSTRUCTIONS

In a food processor or blender, add peanuts and mix. When the blend begins to stick to the sides, turn processor off. Scrape down the sides using a rubber spatula. Repeat process 3–4 times or until you achieve the desired texture for your peanut butter. Add maple syrup, cannabis oil, and sea salt, and process until completely incorporated.

Place banana slices on a heat/oven-safe pan. Coat each slice of banana with 1 Tbsp. of turbinado sugar. Using a kitchen torch, heat the sugar until it is burled.

3 cups of roasted peanuts

4 Tbsp. homemade maple syrup (reference recipe)

½ Tbsp. of cannabis oil
(reference recipe)

¼ tsp. of sea salt

2 bananas (sliced lengthwise)

4 Tbsp. turbinado sugar

One sunny summer morning, my mother declared that we would be taking a trip to the blueberry farm that day. Though tired from an 8-hour drive from Ft. Lauderdale, Florida, to Statesboro, Georgia, the day before, my youthful adrenaline piped up.
I was excited!

We arrived to row upon row of mature blueberry trees brimming with plump ripened fruit—the juicy gates of heaven, in my opinion. My mother gave me a basket to fill and sent me and my sibs off to pick berries, reminding us that we'd pay by the pound. This would have been a good time to weigh the kid (me); before and after!

Row after row, I scoured the trees for the prettiest and plumpest berries. I skipped and grinned with glee. I beckoned my older sister, who on that day was in her "I don't have time for little sisters" mood. I wanted to show her the fruit that I was discovering, to share my happiness. She rebuffed my calls and remained beneath a single tree, harvesting her own share of blueberries.

I shrugged her aloofness off and carried on, happily focused on filling my own basket. But my basket didn't get full as fast as I thought it would. My system appeared to be slightly compromised: one berry for the basket, four berries for Andrea; 10 berries for the basket, 12 for Andrea. By the time we were ready to depart, I looked into my mostly empty basket with dismay. Everyone questioned what I had been doing for the past hour or so. Everyone, including myself! I truly believed that I had divvied up the berries equally between belly and basket. My blue mouth and stained shirt told a different story!

Eventually, of course, the chickens (or should I say the berries) came to roost. I spent the afternoon doubled over in pain and hogging time in the bathroom. I was the butt of many jokes for the rest of the vacation, and though I tried to convince myself that this constituted a food allergy, I would later have to admit to my gluttony when the same thing happened to me after eating a monster quantity of strawberry cake on another occasion. Lucky for me, overindulgence does not equate to food allergies, and it did not destroy my passion for blueberries.

BLUEBERRY SMOOTHIE

YIELDS 4 SERVINGS AT 30 MG PER SERVING

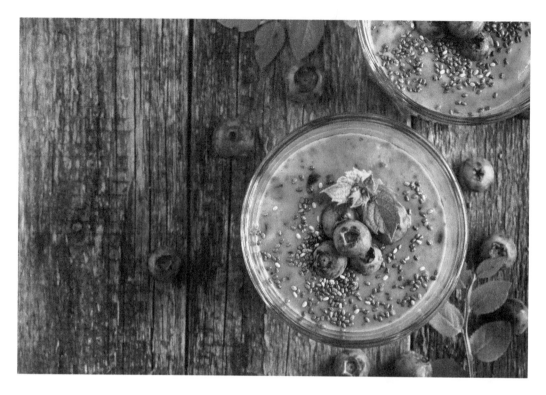

2 cups of infused milk (or almond milk; reference recipe)

2 cups milk

2 cups of fresh blueberries (freeze before using)

2 cups of fresh mango (freeze before using)

2 ounces of hemp seeds

2 Tbsp. of chia seeds

INSTRUCTIONS

In a blender, mix all ingredients until smooth.

CREAM CHEESE GRITS WITH PORK BELLY AND RED EYE GRAVY

YIELDS 8SERVINGS AT 46.5 MG PER SERVING

INGREDIENTS FOR GRAVY:

1 lb. of pork belly (diced)

10 ounces of shallots (diced fine)

2 Tbsp. garlic (minced)

2 sprigs thyme

2 cups of infused coffee (reference recipe)

2 Tbsp. blond roux

10 ounces fire roasted tomatoes
(diced and drained)

8 cups of veal stock

2 ounces balsamic raspberry preserves
(reference recipe)

INGREDIENTS FOR GRITS:

¾ cup of stone ground grits

2 cups vegetable stock
(infused stock optional)

¾ cup heavy cream
(infused heavy cream optional)

5 Tbsp. of cream cheese

4 Tbsp. of pecorino (grated)

INSTRUCTIONS

In a cast iron skillet, cook pork belly over medium low heat until crispy. Remove with slotted spoon and set aside.

Sauté shallots into pork belly fat until soft. Add garlic and thyme until fragrant, but do not let garlic brown. Add tomatoes and cook until soft. Add coffee and continue to cook until it reduces by half. Add the stock and reduce until it is half the original volume. Thicken with the blonde roux. Finish with preserve. Add pork belly back to gravy, and season to taste.

In a medium saucepan, combine vegetable stock, cream, grits, and a pinch of salt. Bring to a boil and reduce to low simmer, stirring frequently. Cook until tender, adding water if needed. Stir in the cream cheese and pecorino. Adjust seasoning to taste.

Divide into 8 servings and serve with pork belly red eye gravy and poached egg.

CONCLUSION

Many years after my 200 completed community hours, I found myself in Brooklyn, New York. By now, I had done extensive work with the Urban League, Planned Parenthood, Coalition for the Homeless and a few other nonprofit entities. Now, however, I was working with a grassroots organization, pushing a gang prevention agenda to junior high and high school aged girls. It was a major adjustment.

Theses beautifully creative and smart young ladies would test you beyond measure. Between Life Skills sessions and day trips to outdoor concerts, they would argue and fight with each other and at times threaten staff. At times, the work was rewarding. But mostly, it was exhausting. This was the first of a number of experiences where I felt that our philosophy was not cohesive and was unfortunately counterproductive. I was burned out and done with being a martyr.

The vibrant language of these evolving young women no longer had a lure. My aspiration to unlock their internal magic had dulled. The labels of promising, at-risk, troubled, or gifted didn't make sense anymore. Were not we all at risk? Don't we all have notable gifts?

One day a "promising" student entered with a new book in tow. She'd gotten it from a book exchange. Its title: Go Ask Alice. What were the chances? This had to be the lifeline that I had hoped for.

Just as it had for me many years previously, the narration of Alice's harrowing experiences beckon the student to dive headlong into the depths of martyrdom. Her declared intention was to become a psychiatrist. I was proud and happy for her.

I shared my own introduction to Go Ask Alice and spoke more about addiction, marijuana, and motivation. "Ms. Andrea, you can borrow it if you want. I'm going out to celebrate my grandmother's birthday, so I won't be doing any reading tonight," she offered. I promised to have it back to her the next day.

I thumbed the pages during the evening, anticipating the second coming of that soul-stirring passion that had led me to here. My fingertips tingled. The anticipation was palpable.

I walked home with it burning my palm. I read while cooking dinner that evening. The television was silenced as I ate and thumbed the tattered pages. I poured a glass of wine and slid under a warm comforter, book in hand. I took in the rhythm of the author; imagined the tone of her voice, and pictured the places she described. I tried to connect to her pain, searching for the jarring nudge that had inspired an entire career. Yet though still softened by the plight of this young woman who would not live to tell a story of redemption, the spell had been broken.

When the last word of the last chapter of the final page was read, I closed the dog-eared paperback and knew instinctually that a chapter in my life, too, had come to an end.

You see, I no longer believed that cannabis was the defining moment for Alice. There were other variables and indicators in her narrative. Life and further experience had revealed that marijuana was frequently the substance easiest to obtain. And often, when it was unable to quiet the hurt, the shift to heavier substances had been a welcomed transition.

I was disconnected from my colleagues and their philosophy. And by now, I had tried cannabis at least 6 times solidly. Though my preference was still a great glass of wine, I no longer harshly judged my friends who smoked with regularity. They would light up, and I would open a dry white wine. Shortly after, someone would be off to the bodega for something fried, sweet, or topped with bacon. I wondered, a gateway to what? Obesity?

A few weeks later, I cued up the computer and fired off. "It is with deep regret that I submit my letter of resignation..." My rebirth had begun.

I am not a hippie but a self-professed tree hugger. I did not live in San Francisco when cannabis was called dope. Nor did I traipse the streets of Venice when Basquiat could have been blocks away. It was a time when a stoic Nancy Reagan encouraged drug-free contracts between parents and children, and we eagerly believed in their value. I am from a religious upbringing that condemned any drug that was not prescribed by the almighty physician. In a complete 360, my belief now is that food and cannabis are both medicine.

Through this culinary journey, I hope that you have gained a sense of cannabis cookery as well as the journey that led me here. It is important to me that you've learned the basic skills to properly integrate microdosing and cannabis cuisine adequately into a routine that works for your purpose. Have fun with cooking, and integrate yourself in a way that nourishes your body medicinally and otherwise.

QUICK REFERENCE

CANNABIS INFUSED BUTTERMILK

YIELDS 1 QUART AT 50 MG OF THC PER CUP

1 quart buttermilk

1 cup water

2 gram sachet of cannabis product

INSTRUCTIONS

In a saucepan, bring the buttermilk and water to a boil. Add the sachet of cannabis and lower the heat. Allow to simmer for 40 minutes. Stir occasionally to assure that the milk does not scald. Remove from heat, cool, squeeze out sachet and discard.

*Product can also be used for pancakes, biscuits etc.

** Recipes based on product containing 10% THC

INFUSED HEAVY CREAM

YIELDS 4 CUPS AT 120 MG PER SERVING

4 cups heavy cream

2 grams cannabis in a sachet

INSTRUCTIONS

Place cream in saucepan with sachet and heat on very low temperature for 30 minutes. Allow to cool and squeeze sachet. Place cream in container and use as needed.

VEGETABLE STOCK

YIELDS 2 QUARTS (64 CUPS) AT 1.7 MG OF THC PER 1 CUP

2 large onions (quartered)

2 leeks (chopped)

5 celery stalks (chopped)

2 large carrots (peeled and chopped)

1 Tbsp. olive oil

5 ounces crimini mushrooms

2 bay leaves

1 sprig rosemary

4 sprigs of thyme

2 1½ cups white port wine

1 head of garlic (halved)

1 fennel bulb (chopped)

1 tsp. whole black peppercorns

1 Tbsp. tomato paste

½ gram sachet of cannabis product

INSTRUCTIONS

Heat the oil in a large stockpot over medium-high heat. Add all ingredients except sachet, tomato paste, wine, and water. Cook until the vegetables begin to soften.

Add the tomato paste and cook until it begins to slightly caramelize (darken). Deglaze the vegetables with the port wine. Cook until the wine reduces. Add 4 quarts of cold water and bring to a boil, then reduce to low simmer until the stock is reduced by half, 1–1½ hours.

Strain stock through a fine-mesh sieve into a large bowl, pressing to release all of the liquids. Discard solids. Freeze and use as needed.

DO AHEAD: Stock can be made 3 days ahead. Let cool completely, then cover and chill, or freeze for up to 3 months.

MUSHROOM STOCK

YIELDS 2 QUARTS (64 CUPS) AT 3.43 MG OF THC PER 1 CUP

1 large yellow onion (quartered)

2 cups mushroom stems

2 ounces dried shitake mushrooms

1 cup fresh assorted mushroom tops

1 leek (chopped)

1 head of garlic (halved)

1 bay leaf

2 celery stalks

1 tsp. peppercorns

1 gram sachet of cannabis material

2 Tbsp. roasted garlic cannabis oil (reference recipe)

1 ½ cup dry white wine

4 quarts of water

INSTRUCTIONS

Heat roasted garlic cannabis oil in a stockpot. Add onions, chopped celery, peppercorns, leek, and bay leaf. Cook until onion is translucent. Add head of garlic, and cook for another 4 minutes. Increase the heat and add mushroom stems, shitake mushrooms, and assorted mushroom tops. Cook another 3 minutes. Deglaze with white wine and lower the heat. Allow the wine to reduce. Add 4 quarts of cold water, bring to a boil, then reduce to low simmer until the stock is reduced by half. Strain, pressing out as much liquid as possible

Cool in an ice bath. Freeze and use as needed.

*Recipes based on product containing 22% THC

PASTA DOUGH

YIELDS 7 1-OUNCE SERVINGS OF DOUGH AT 5 MG PER SERVING

6 ounces Tipo 00 Italian flour

2 ounces all-purpose flour

3 medium egg yolks

1 medium egg

1 ¼ cup water

1 cup balsamic vinegar

¼ tsp. cannabis oil (reference recipe)

½ Tbsp. water

INSTRUCTIONS

Sift Tipo and all-purpose flour. Add into mixer. Turn mixer on low and add egg yolks one at a time. Then add the full egg. Mix on low and slowly add the cannabis oil. Add water.

Mix until ball forms. Add additional all-purpose flour in small amounts if needed. Knead the dough on lightly floured surface. Cover in plastic wrap and refrigerate for at least 30 minutes.

Portion the dough into 1-ounce balls. Roll out using a pasta machine.

INFUSED MAYONNAISE

YIELDS 12 SERVINGS AT 11.7 MG PER SERVING

1 large egg yolk

1 ½ tsp. fresh lemon juice

1 tsp. white wine vinegar

¼ tsp. Dijon mustard

½ tsp. salt plus more to taste

11 Tbsp. California olive oil, divided

1 Tbsp. infused cannabis oil (reference recipe)

INSTRUCTIONS

Combine egg yolk, lemon juice, vinegar, mustard, and ½ tsp. salt in medium bowl. Whisk until blended and bright yellow, about 30 seconds. Using quarter tsp. measure and whisking constantly, add ¼ cup oil (combine 1 Tbsp. cannabis oil and 3 Tbsp. olive oil) to yolk mixture a few drops at a time, over about 4 minutes. Gradually add remaining half cup of olive oil in a very slow thin stream, whisking constantly, until mayonnaise is thick, about 8 minutes (mayonnaise will be lighter in color). Cover and chill.

BLUEBERRY BBQ SAUCE

YIELDS 8 SERVINGS AT 2 OUNCES AND 18.75 MG PER SERVING

2 cups fresh blueberries

1 can tomato sauce

½ cup balsamic vinegar

⅓ cup honey

¼ cup tomato paste

¼ cup molasses

3 Tbsp. Worcestershire sauce

2 tsp. liquid smoke

1 tsp. smoked paprika

2 cloves minced garlic

½ tsp. black pepper

½ tsp. onion powder

½ tsp. salt

1 Tbsp. cannabis oil (reference recipe)

INSTRUCTIONS

Whisk all ingredients together in medium saucepan. Bring to simmer over medium-high heat. Reduce heat to medium low and simmer uncovered for 20 minutes, or until the sauce has thickened. Place in blender and blend until smooth.

PIE CRUST

2 ½ cups all-purpose flour

1 tsp. salt

2 Tbsp. sugar

¾ cup (a stick and a half) unsalted butter, chilled, cut into ¼-inch cubes

½ cup of all-vegetable shortening (8 Tbsp.)

6–8 Tbsp. ice water

INSTRUCTIONS

Combine flour, salt, and sugar in a food processor; pulse to mix. Add the butter and pulse 4 times. Add shortening in Tbsp. sized chunks, and pulse 4 more times. The mixture should resemble coarse cornmeal, with butter bits no bigger than peas. Sprinkle 6 Tbsp. of ice water over flour mixture. Pulse a couple of times. If you pinch some of the crumbly dough and it holds together, it's ready. If the dough doesn't hold together, keep adding water, a Tbsp. at a time, pulsing once after each addition, until the mixture just begins to clump together.

Remove dough from machine and place in a mound on a clean surface. Divide the dough into 2 balls, and flatten each into 4-inch wide disks. Do not over-knead the dough! Dust the disks lightly with flour, wrap each in plastic, and refrigerate for at least an hour, or up to 2 days before rolling out.

After the dough has chilled in the refrigerator for an hour, you can take it out to roll. If it is too stiff, you may need to let it sit for 5–10 minutes at room temperature before rolling. Sprinkle a little flour on a flat, clean work surface and on top of the disk of dough you intend to roll out.

CURRY PASTE

YIELDS 8 SERVINGS AT 12.5 MG PER SERVING

2 tsp. coriander seeds

1 tsp. dry mustard

½ tsp. cumin

8 whole black peppercorns

2 Tbsp. cilantro (rough chopped)

2 tsp. shrimp paste

1½ tsp. kosher salt

1 tsp. ground Kaffir lime leaves

1 tsp. grated lime zest

4 fresh green Thai chilies

6 cloves garlic (rough chopped)

6 small Asian shallots or 2 medium regular shallots (sliced thin)

1½ stalks lemongrass (trimmed and sliced thin)

6"piece galangal (peeled and sliced thin)

4" ginger (peeled and minced)

1 gram ground cannabis

INSTRUCTIONS

Make the paste: Heat coriander seeds, dry mustard, cumin, and peppercorns in a cast-iron skillet until seeds begin to pop, 1–2 minutes. Let it cool, and place in spice grinder and pulse until finely ground. Set aside until you complete the next steps.

Place cilantro root, shrimp paste, salt, kaffir lime leaves, lime zest, chilies, garlic, shallots, lemongrass, and galangal in a small food processor; pulse until roughly chopped. Add spice mixture.

LOBSTER STOCK

YIELDS 2 QUARTS (64 CUPS) SERVINGS AT 3.43 MG PER 1 CUP

Shells and heads from 4 cooked lobsters

2 large peeled carrots (rough chopped)

2 large onions (rough chopped)

4 Tbsp. tomato paste

1 head of garlic (halved horizontally)

8 Tbsp. of butter

1 Tbsp. black peppercorns

2 sprigs of thyme

1 bay leaf

1 sprig of tarragon

1 bunch of parsley

2 cups of dry white wine

1 cup of Madeira wine

12 cups of water

1 gram sachet of cannabis

INSTRUCTIONS

In a larger stockpot, heat butter and Tbsp. of olive oil. Add shells and let cook for 3–5 minutes, allowing butter to fortify with the seafood flavor. Add onion, carrots, and garlic, and cook until onions are soft, stirring frequently. Add tomato paste, stir until vegetables and shells are coated. Add the herbs and pepper corn. Cook for 3 minutes. Deglaze with the white wine and reduce. Add the Madeira and cannabis and cook for additional 3–5 minutes. Add water and lower heat to simmer uncovered. Cook until it reduces to about half (8 cups). Strain in freezer safe container and use as needed.

You can substitute ½ tsp. cannabis butter for a sachet of cannabis (yields slightly higher potency of 4.4 mg per cup of stock)

INFUSED MILK

YIELDS 4 CUPS AT 120 MG PER 1 CUP SERVING

4 cups milk

1 gram cannabis in a sachet

INSTRUCTIONS

Place milk in saucepan with sachet and heat on very low temperature for 30 minutes. Allow to cool, and squeeze sachet. Place milk in container and use as needed.

INFUSED ALMOND MILK

YIELDS 4 CUPS AT 60 MG PER 1 CUP SERVING

4 cups almond milk

1 gram cannabis in a satchet

INSTRUCTIONS

Place milk in saucepan with sachet and heat on very low temperature for 30 minutes. Allow to cool and squeeze sachet. Place milk in container and use as needed.

ELEVATED FIVE-SPICE SEASONING

YIELDS 11 (TSP.) SERVINGS AT 21 MG PER SERVING

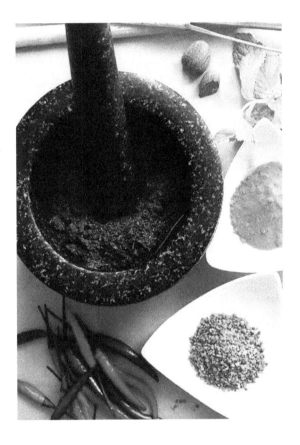

2 Tbsp. dry star anise (ground)

2 Tbsp. fennel seed (ground)

2 tsp. cinnamon (ground)

2 tsp. Szechuan pepper corn (ground)

¼ tsp. cloves (ground)

1 tsp. cannabis (ground)

PORK BELLY REDEYE GRAVY

YIELDS 8 SERVINGS AT 46.5 MG PER SERVING

1 lb. of pork belly diced

10 ounces of shallots (diced fine)

2 Tbsp. garlic (minced)

2 sprigs thyme

2 cups of infused coffee (reference recipe)

2 Tbsp. blond roux

10 ounces fire roasted tomatoes (diced and drained)

8 cups of veal stock

2 ounces balsamic raspberry preserves (reference recipe)

INSTRUCTIONS

In a cast iron skillet, cook pork belly over medium low heat until crispy. Remove with slotted spoon and set aside.

Sautee shallots into pork belly fat until soft. Add garlic and thyme until fragrant, but do not let garlic brown. Add tomatoes and cook until soft. Add coffee until it reduces by half. Add the stock and reduce until only half the original volume remains. Thicken with the blonde roux. Finish with preserve. Add pork belly back to gravy and season to taste.

HOLLANDAISE SAUCE

YIELDS 6 SERVINGS AT 11.6 MG PER SERVING

½ cup clarified butter

1 tsp. clean cannabis butter (reference recipe)

3 egg yolks

2 tsp. lemon juice

½ tsp. cayenne pepper

½ tsp. Dijon mustard

Kosher salt to taste

Melt the butter in a small saucepan over low heat. Place the egg yolks, cayenne, mustard, and lemon juice into a blender. Blend until the mixture is foamy and slightly stiffened.

With the blender running, gradually add the clarified butter in a thin stream. Season to taste with kosher salt.

The sauce should be served within an hour. Keep in a warm spot.

POACHED EGGS

Heat a pot of water to a bare simmer. Crack an egg into a small bowl or ramekin, and gently slip the egg into the water. Do this for each egg. Turn off the heat, cover the pot, and let sit for 4 minutes or until egg whites are solid. Gently remove eggs with slotted spoon. Place on top of toasted English muffin, spoon hollandaise over the egg; serve with your favorite cocktail.

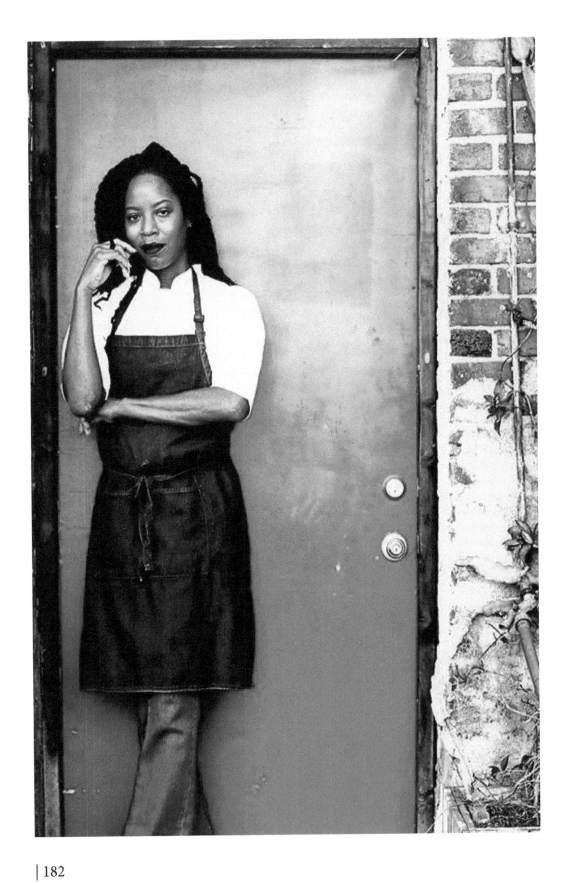

AUTHOR BIO

Chef Andrea Drummer began her career, first as a youth advocate and anti-drug counselor with organizations like Planned Parenthood and The Coalition for the Homeless. With a desire to transition from the world of non-profit to pursue her passion, she enrolled at Le Cordon Bleu, Los Angeles. This second career found her working at the renowned Ritz Carlton and with the likes of famed Chef Neal Frazer. The two worlds would oddly collide as Chef Drummer deepened her understanding of the schedule 1 drug that she had once advocated so vehemently against. In 2012, she co-founded Elevation VIP Cooperative and become versed in cooking with cannabis. A staunch advocate for the legalization of marijuana, Chef Drummer has gained a wealth of knowledge working with local activists and allies while cooking for the likes of Chelsea Handler and other noted celebrities. She has been featured in Marie Claire Magazine, Vogue Online, Pop-Sugar, 60 Second Docs and LA Times and was recently named 1 of 10 Top Cannabis Chefs in the country. As an entrepreneur and a patient, she continues to spread her new gospel about the benefits of cannabis by educating, advocating and cooking.

Thank you Lowell Farms for sponsoring a phenomenal product that inspires me to create. Yours is the Aston Martin of the cannabis industry. Lowellsmokes.com

Thanks to the supporters, activists, advocates and true believers; I am inspired by your fight.

Thank you to Hamady Diallo and Nickole Ross for your unwavering love and support. You make me better.

Printed in the USA
CPSIA information can be obtained
at www.ICGtesting.com
JSHW072019140824
68134JS00040B/3705